Herbal Apothecary

The Best Herbal Medicine and How to Grow and Use to Self Healing

author of this work can be in any fashion deemed liable for any hardship or damages that may befall them after undertaking information described herein.

Additionally, the information in the following pages is intended only for informational purposes and should thus be thought of as universal. As befitting its nature, it is presented without assurance regarding its prolonged validity or interim quality. Trademarks that are mentioned are done without written consent and can in no way be considered an endorsement from the trademark holder.

Table of Contents

Introduction

Congratulations on downloading *Herbal Apothecary* and thank you for doing so.

The following chapters will discuss herbs that you can grow in your garden that have some medicinal benefits and those that can possibly help alleviate some issues that are relatively common, and maybe some other issues that are not so common. In addition to providing information about the herbs, information on proper drying, gardening, and storage of herbs are also included. The use of herbs in treating ailments dates back thousands of years and has been a tradition for several cultures around the world, but information on their use how to grow them and how to ensure home-grown quality can be difficult to find. With the vast number of supplements available in your local vitamin store and online, it can be overwhelming for someone new to alternative healthcare. Sometimes, you just don't know where to start.

There are plenty of books on this subject on the market, thanks again for choosing this one! Every effort was made to ensure it is full of as much useful information as possible, please enjoy!

Chapter 1: The History of Herbal Medicine

From several various sources, we can trace man's use of plants and herbs for medicine as far back as mankind itself. In fact, a number of drugs on the market today are based in folk medicine from the herbal world. Herbal medicines are made from whole plants or parts of a plant. Also known as botanical medicines, supplements or sometimes remedies. Although these types of treatments are becoming more integrated into main-stream medical treatments, typically herbal medicine has been a self-treatment route for minor symptoms and non-life-threatening diseases. However, a lot of the drugs available on the market for treatment and alleviation of pain, are based on herbal or botanical materials. Examples of these are: aspirin, digitalis, atropine, morphine, quinine, and more. Research is happening every day to take what nature has done and extract the benefits

Some of the oldest written evidence of herbal medicine can be dated back to Sumeria about 5000 years ago. The Chinese had a book of 365 herbal medicine that was used around 2500 BC. The Ebers Papyrus, written around 1550 BC, is a collection of applications of herbal medicine representing about 700 plant species including Aloe Vera, castor oil, pomegranate, willow, fig, garlic, juniper, and more. Before the sixteenth century, a common practice in healing was to use the body's ability to heal itself and to supplement that with the right herbs. Monasteries traditionally had entire gardens devoted to growing the type of herbs that could be used to treat the public because healing was included in the responsibilities of the religious people. The monks were generally more educated than the general public, so they gathered information on the correct cultivating and harvesting practices, beneficial properties of the herb, as well as having access to importing plants not native to the area. This allowed them to expand their repertoire of treatments available.

One of the quintessential sources on herbal medicine, Culpeper's *The Complete Herbal*, was published in 1649 and has gone through over 100 editions. Since Culpeper was British, he focused on British plants and published his guide in English so that the reference guide could be of use to the public (at the time most reference guides were published in Latin, but Culpeper felt this would greatly reduce the audience of the guide). Although his guide was incredibly useful, it angered the medical establishments because herbal apothecaries were sometimes the more affordable healthcare for the general public, thus the doctors thought it was stealing their business. Unfortunately, Culpeper died at the age of 38 from tuberculosis.

As society progressed out of the Middle Ages, new plants from the Americas became known and their benefits were discovered and integrated into use as well. Over the next century, gardening radically changed as a number of new plants and seeds were discovered and brought back to be cultivated into main-stream usage. One of the first botanical gardens used for studying the plants was established at Oxford in 1621. It allowed the study of the use of herbs as medicinal treatments. This paved the way for herbs to enter the mainstream market and accelerated the spread of their health benefits to doctors and to the public.

In recent years, herbal healing has seen a new rise in popularity given the new age culture and interest in "alternative" or "holistic" medicine. Herbal treatments allow the public to essentially participate in their own self-care and keep treatments on a more natural basis. Although there are more references now about herbal medicines than 60 years ago, it is still worth the time of consumers to do a little homework before investing in supplements or other holistic treatments. Supplements are not regulated in the same way as traditional pharmaceutical medicines, so there might be a lot of products on the market that are not of the best quality and are not the most effective treatment for your ailment. With supplements, the quality and quantity can make a big difference as can the application; taking a supplement versus consuming an herbal tea can have a different effect—so it pays to be informed. And this may drive some followers of alternative medicine to pursue growing and dispensing the herbs themselves. In order for this to be the best experience, the consumer needs to understand each herb or plant, how it is best used (tincture, tea, supplement, poultice, etc.), the growing conditions, time of harvest, the manner of extraction, the manner of preparation and other details.

Note: All herbs should be used with caution because they contain powerful bioactive compounds. Start with small quantities initially to test your tolerance. Watch out for allergic reactions. People who have ragweed allergy may have similar reactions to medicinal plants belonging to that family.

When you feel good with a recommended amount of a given herb, it doesn't necessarily mean that you will feel better with larger quantities or a stronger brew. To derive maximum benefit out of the herbs you grow, try to learn as much about them as you can.

Chapter 2: Easy Herbs to Grow in Your Garden

There are a number of people with green thumbs who are capable of growing anything. But for those that struggle to make a flower bloom, there is still hope that you can grow, will flourish, and can then be used at home to the best benefits.

1.   **<u>Alfalfa</u>** (*Medicago sativa*):

Although alfalfa is an herb, most people are familiar with it as a primary food source for farm animals. Which actually makes sense because alfalfa is recognized as one of the most nutritious food forages available. For humans, that holds true in addition to a number of actual health benefits. One of the reasons alfalfas rank is so high on the list of beneficial herbs is because the body can easily absorb and put the nutrients found in this plant to use. Alfalfa can help with a lot of issues like nausea, urinary tract problems (prostate, infections, or kidney stones), cleansing of toxins found in the liver, cholesterol, allergies, tooth decay, milk supply for nursing, cleans the blood, blood clotting, pituitary gland, blood sugar levels, and more. Combined with sage, it may even ease menopause symptoms as it boosts the pituitary. It is a good daily source of minerals like iron, potassium, calcium, sulfur, phosphorous, and magnesium and vitamins A, C, E and K4. In addition, there are a number of essential amino acids that the body doesn't produce on its own, so we must get them from food. Alfalfa is a good source of these essential amino acids. If you are a fan of the green powders available for morning smoothies, alfalfa is frequently used as a base ingredient of those because it is so easy to use and digest, and it contains high chlorophyll contents.

Alfalfa is a perennial crop that is a good cover crop or soil conditioner. If you have a spot in your garden that seems soil depleted, plant alfalfa in that corner for a year or two. It is a drought resistant plant. In fact, it doesn't like being too wet for that can lead to mold growth. Choose an area with a lot of all-day sun and proper drainage. They do not require deep planting and the form roots rather quickly. Sow the seeds about one-half inch (.5") deep and cover lightly. Sprouts will appear in about 7-10 days. Thin the seeds as needed to give them a little growing room. Harvest for use before the purple blooms appear.

If you plan to grow alfalfa indoors, you can easily use a small jar or pot base and produce a much smaller crop. One tablespoon of seeds will produce about 1.5 cups of alfalfa. Wash the seeds you plan to use and remove any broken or discolored seeds. Place the washed seeds into a glass quart jar. Cover the prepared seeds with about two (2) inches of cold water; make sure they are completely covered. Do not use a metal lid but cover the jar with a small piece of cheesecloth; you can secure with a rubber band to keep the cloth tight. Keep the jar in a warm place for about 12 hours. Filtered sunlight is helpful, but direct sunlight is not necessary. Drain the water, rinse, and drain again. Tilt the jar on its side and place in a dark location that is warm. Spread the seeds out. Rinse the seeds again every 8-12 hours, draining well after each rinse. Do this for about four (4) days or until the seeds sprout and are about two (2) inches long. Spread the sprouts out into a thin layer on a flat surface and put them in a sunny location, wait for about 15 minutes for the leaves to turn green and the enzymes to activate. Now they're ready to be used on salads, sandwiches, or just to snack on.

A great alternative is to use the base of a clay pot; spread the soaked seeds on this base and put the base into a larger, shallow container of water. The clay will absorb enough water to keep the seeds hydrated. Make sure you use quality water and it will keep the plants as nutritional as possible. If you want to remove the coats from the sprouts, you just need to put them in a bowl of water and agitate the water briefly. The seed coats float to the top and you can take them out, leaving the hulled sprouts behind. You can use the sprouts fresh or keep them in the refrigerator.

Alfalfa is typically grown for feed or for use in the kitchen, it is not typically used as a decorative, flowering plant.

2.   <u>Aloe Vera</u> (*A. barbadensis* Mill.)**:**

This plant has a history of being a go-to source for treating burns and skin irritation when applied topically. However, aloe can also act as a helpful laxative when consumed and, in fact, has a myriad of healing properties. It has antibacterial, antifungal, and antiviral properties. It also can be used to relax the bowels and alleviate stomachaches.

For home use, it is generally safe and requires no processing before use. Aloe can be grown in almost any garden, either in pots or in the ground. They do well in a sunny location and in warm areas where frost wouldn't be an issue. It is a member of the succulent family, so it is drought resistant and it requires little watering, little care, and can thrive even in poor soil. Although there are several varieties of aloe, make sure you get Aloe Vera to ensure you get a plant with medicinal properties that would be edible.

When you have a burn, aloe can be a quick treatment. Snap off a piece and use the jelly-like, colorless pulp to smear onto the burn. This acts as an anti-inflammatory and antimicrobial ointment. It is incredibly easy to use it for consumption as well. Wash the Aloe Vera leaf, cut it open, and scoop out the gel (gel should be clear; discard any greenish gel). Store the aloe in a glass jar and refrigerate for use. Add 2 teaspoons of gel to filtered water or any type of fruit juice. Regular ingestion can help prevent or relieve constipation and other digestive problems, which can include ulcerative colitis and irritable bowel syndrome.

Aloe Vera plants can be really carefree house plants. They can be grown indoors in pots even without a green thumb. The soil should be allowed to dry in between watering to discourage rot. Water the plant approximately every 21 days but even more sparingly during the winter. This plant does not require a lot of fertilizer. You may put fertilizer for no more than once a month only in spring and summer. It will probably need repotting when it becomes root bound and use a potting soil specifically developed for succulents.

Aloe Vera can be an attractive succulent grown in houseplants on the kitchen windowsill. With its long, slender, star-like appearance, it can add some pretty greenery to any corner.

3.   **<u>Cayenne</u>** (*Capsicum annuum*):

This is a hemostatic herb that can help to stop bleeding. It might be an organic substitute for a baby aspirin to slow the progression of a heart attack. In addition, cayenne may serve to boost metabolism as it raises the amount of heat your body produces so that you naturally burn more calories in a day. A small boost, but when dieting and watching calories, every little bit of assistance can help. Some studies show that the capsaicin may also help to reduce hunger, which further helps to reduce the amount of caloric intake every day.

This well-known addition to your diet may even help

to reduce high blood pressure, although current research has only been conducted with animals. Cayenne may also benefit your stomach in a way that isn't just good tasting, as it may actually boost the enzymes in your stomach which aid in digestion. Contrary to popular belief which warns against consuming spicy foods, cayenne may actually serve as a protection against ulcers. Capsaicin is also a common ingredient in most muscle rubs and creams that help to reduce aches and soreness. The symptoms of Psoriasis, an autoimmune disease that manifests in patches of scaly and red skin, can sometimes be alleviated by capsaicin.

A lot of people grow a variety of peppers in their garden and for good reason. They are easy to grow and easy to use. Chilies are sub-tropical and mostly perennial and they like heat. If you live in a climate that is consistently warm enough, plant them outside. Otherwise, you can put them in a pot and bring them indoors when necessary. Seeds should be planted in a sunny location in soil that drains well. If planting outside, seeds should be initially planted inside and transferred outdoors. Generally, transplanting should occur about seven (7) weeks after the seeds are sown. Moist soil is required, but take care not to add too much water.

Peppers are typically added to a garden for the produce; not for appearance. However, the plants themselves can be quite beautiful with their shocking red peppers. In fact, a number of ornamental peppers plants have been marketed just because of the appearance. This can add a bright splash of color to any kitchen.

2. Chamomile (*Chamaemelum nobile*):

With a lovely scent, this herb is most well known as a tea for relaxation. Most people drink it at the end of the day to calm down, ease stress, and some women use it to relieve menstrual cramps. In addition, it can be used to soothe a baby crying from colic. A tincture from flowers can also be used as a gargle to help with canker or mouth ulcers. People who suffer from eczema can use the cooled tea as a compress to ease symptoms. An anti-inflammatory, chamomile is less commonly used to treat digestive issues, improve the function of the liver, cleanse the blood, treat skin blisters, alleviate arthritis pain, and boost the pancreas. Drinking chamomile tea at night will promote a more restful sleep. The most effective and useful type is the Roman chamomile. The daisy type of flowers is a pretty addition to pots or a garden as well.

In the garden, sow the seeds in the Spring or Fall as chamomile prefers cool soil. It needs light, so scatter the seeds, but do not bury in the soil. Place them in an area that is full sun. Mature plants should be ready for use in about 90 days. Although you can get a jumpstart if you establish plants from another plant rather than from seeds. Once established, it takes very little care, as do most herbs. The herb is drought tolerant. It's a good plant to put around the outside of a garden as the potent scent can sometimes keep pests away.

Chamomile is a beautiful, flowering plant and if you are fond of daisies, you will be fond of seeing this sprouting in your backyard as well. With the cluster of small white flowers and relaxing smell, this is a definite bonus for any edging, garden, or flower bed.

3.   **Dandelion** (*Taraxacum*):

Another weed that is super simple to grow and most people do so without ever intending to. It's good for treating liver and kidney issues as it's a diuretic in addition to supporting digestion and promoting hormone health. As the plant is edible, it's easy to add the greens to salads or to make a tea from the flowers. Dandelion is a good source of a variety of nutrients, and the leaves and roots contain vitamins like A, C, K and B-vitamins as well as minerals including magnesium, zinc, potassium, iron, calcium, and choline. Other parts of the plant can be used in various herbal remedies and almost every lawn has these flowers popping up. While you can put the leaves into a salad, you can brew the flowers into tea or even into wine (although that has fewer health benefits). Since the dandelion is high in zinc and magnesium, it can be used to treat skin conditions.

Almost everyone from a child to grandpa can recognize a dandelion flower. Those bright yellow heads that poke up in early spring. Most people who take care of a yard can rolls their eyes and sigh when seeing a sea of yellow starting to spread across the yard. But those plants should be a welcome sight to anyone using herbal medicine and natural teas.

4. **<u>Echinacea</u>** (*Echinacea purpurea*)**:**

Echinacea is a steadfast staple in native North American herbal medicine. It helps the body fight both bacterial and viral infections. The fields across America host an array of flowers, some just pretty and some pretty useful. Echinacea, or the purple coneflower (*Echinacea purpurea*), is one of the best. Historically, Native Americans used the roots to treat a variety of issues from an insect bite to a snake bite. More recently, the flower buds have made their way into alternative treatments for a cold or the flu. A tincture made with alcohol is considered more potent; steep the flower buds or roots, or both, in pure, concentrated alcohol for 4-6 weeks, and then filter out the liquid. Echinacea is believed to be a natural defense mechanism that boosts the white blood cells, assisting your body in combating infections and bacteria.

Most commonly, Echinacea is grown best outside in a garden. Plants bloom heavily from July through September and can make your garden a haven for both butterflies and bees. Standing tall at 3-4 feet, they make a bright, eye-catching border. To thrive, plants should be planted in full sun, in a rich soil with good drainage because they only require a small amount of water but they will endure most conditions. These biennial plants flower only in the second season. To extend the blooming season, pinch off finished flowers on a regular basis.

With the pastel flowers of Echinacea, it is a welcome addition to your backyard. The daisy shaped flowers have a high, spiky seed cone and last about a month when they bloom. This can add a nice splash of color and pleasing aroma to any flower bed.

5.   **Garlic** (*Allium sativum*):

Garlic is a well-known herb when it comes to both heart health and cooking. A member of the onion family, it is closely related to leeks, shallots, and onions. As is it so prevalent in cooking, the use of garlic for medicinal and health benefits goes back into ancient history. Perhaps the most beneficial elements of garlic are the sulfur compounds that are released, however, this means that ingestion must occur shortly after it is crushed. Garlic is an anti-bacterial, anti-parasitic, and anti-septic that can help purify the blood and promote healthy circulation. It may also help to balance blood sugar levels. In addition to the medicinal benefits, garlic contains a number of vitamins and minerals (B6, C, manganese, selenium) but very few calories. Regular usage of garlic as a supplement has been shown to boost your immune system and lower high blood pressure and cholesterol levels. In addition, studies suggest that it is a powerful antioxidant. Historically, garlic has been used by athletes in the Olympic games of ancient Greece to reduce fatigue and boost energy. The sulfur compounds in garlic may also help to protect against organ damage from heavy metal toxicity. Garlic has also been used as an ingredient in remedies for yeast infections, heart problems, asthma and sinus infections, and to fight bone loss.

Growing your own garlic may be one of the easiest home gardening projects. Softneck bulbs are typically found in most grocery stores and are the easiest to grow in mild regions. If you are planting inside, this is the type of bulb you would probably choose. If you are planting outdoors, you can choose softneck if you are in a mild climate. But may want to choose hardnecks if you have a real winter as they may not produce sufficient bulbs in warm climates. You may also want to choose the hardneck variety because you can also use their flower buds (scapes) as greens. For outdoors, planting usually occurs in mid-fall. Cloves should be inserted root-side down, spacing them at around eight (8) inches apart, and burying them about two (2) inches down. The bulbs are ready for harvesting when the lower leaves have browned but the upper leaves still look green. Gently remove the bulbs from the soil. If you are planting indoors or in a container, make sure that the bulb has plenty of room to spread out. The container should be placed in a spot that gets at least 6 hours of direct sunlight per day. Make sure the container drains well. Again, they should be harvested gently, and the bulbs can then be used in a variety of cooking or eaten raw for health benefits. However, as a daily supplement, it is best to obtain quality capsules from your local reputable health food or vitamin shop.

6. **<u>Ginger</u>** (*Zingiber officinale*):

Ginger is a popular treatment for an upset stomach; it slows the production of serotonin, a chemical trigger for nausea. It can stop vomiting and alleviate general nausea and motion sickness. It is also used to treat indigestion and circulatory problems. Chewing raw ginger or drinking a tea made from ginger or containing ginger can help. Ginger is a natural ingredient that can be an effective weapon in the fight against morning sickness since it is safe to use even during pregnancy. Ginger tea can also help when suffering from a cold or the flu. Ginger promotes sweating and warms the body from within allowing it to alleviate fever or chills. In addition, ginger may be helpful in reducing inflammation, pain associated with a menstrual cycle, cholesterol, risk of blood clotting, and high sugar levels in the blood.

To make ginger tea at home, simply slice about 30 grams of fresh ginger and steep it in hot water for a few minutes. You can add a slice of lemon to boost vitamin C levels as well or add honey for a little sweetness.

As long as you remember that ginger is a tropical plant and it likes hot and humid areas, it is easy to grow your own ginger in your kitchen. Start with a living ginger root. Select a root with tight skin that is firm and plump. Root should have several eye buds as well. Soak the ginger root in warm water overnight to prepare for planting. Since the roots will grow horizontally, choose a wide, shallow pot and fill it with well-draining potting soil. Insert the ginger root with the eye bud pointing up and cover it with 1-2 inches more of soil. Water the root lightly. Make sure the pot stays warm and doesn't get a lot of bright light, keep the soil moist, but not soaking wet. This is a slow process, so it may take 2-3 weeks before you see shoots coming up.

7.   **<u>Great Mullein</u>** (*Verbascum thapsus*):

The medicinal benefits of mullein can date back to the early American settlers who brought it over from Europe because of it capability help treat various ailments like diarrhea and coughs. The utilization of the plant as medicinal treatment spread from the settlers to the Native Americans. Both the flowers and leaves can be used in various treatments, primarily related to respiratory tract problems. Tea made from the leaves and flowers can be used as an expectorant to relieve coughs associated with ailments such as bronchitis. Believe it or not, smoking the mullein leaves has been used to relieve chest congestion as the plant helps to loosen phlegm and flush out the lungs.

Some of the potential benefits of mullein are for the following: warts, athlete's foot, cough, skin infections, sore throat, asthma, bronchitis, and more. You can crush the mullein flowers to make a paste, put it on a wound and it will work as an antiseptic. It also has antiviral properties that may help to ease symptoms associated with a viral infection. Drinking mullein tea may also help to reduce bad cholesterol levels which reduces the risk of high blood pressure and other heart diseases. Extract from the flower can be added to hair rinses to help keep the scalp healthy, stop dandruff, and will naturally enhance your hair's color.

Even if you have very little gardening experience, mullein is a great plant to start with because it is easy to grow and maintain. Since it is classified as a weed, the plant thrives almost anywhere. Place seeds about 18 inches apart in a garden bed on top of the soil. The area should have good drainage because mullein doesn't like excessively moist soil. If possible, plant in an area with access to direct sunlight. The plants need very little watering; never keep the soil soggy. Definitely, give them room as the stalks can grow for as long as seven (7) feet tall.

Make sure you remove the rosettes as they grow, or you will have all the seeds (100,000+) sowing on the wind where they can lay dormant for many years. If multiple rosettes form and all those seeds spread and then grow, you might end up with a big mullein population on your hands.

With pretty yellow flowers and fuzzy leaves, this plant can make a great border, but make sure you plant them in the back as they can grow taller than some people.

8.   **<u>Lavender</u>** (*Lavandula*):

The herb is known as a natural stress reliever and is used prominently in relaxation and sleep applications. In the market, there are a ton of lavender scented candles, lavender essential oil, and teas that are to be used at bedtime to help those suffering from insomnia to nod off. Furthermore, lavender can be used as a treatment for burns and as an antiseptic. For example, if you soak some flowers in water, you can then use that water to wash your face and it may help treat acne.

It can be a great addition to a garden or pots on the patio since bees love them and their flowers smell wonderful. Lavender can be grown in both gardens and in pots, but they are most impressive in a field where they can spread and cover the ground. It needs full sun and well-drained soil to grow best. Lavender is hardy, but in hot summer climates, afternoon shade may help it thrive more. Slightly alkaline soils will produce the best results.

There are pictures all over the internet showing the beauty of lavender fields. Awash with the purple color, these stand out as an oasis of beauty. But you can have a similar corner in your backyard by planting these blooming beauties that will release such a fragrance that when you visit that corner of your garden, you will simply breathe deeply and sigh.

9.   **<u>Lemon Balm</u>** (*Melissa officinalis*):

Lemon balm is a member of the mint family. This lemon-scented herb can be found in oil, extract, salve, or tincture form. It is known to help ease anxiety and stress and is often used for insomnia. In addition, it has benefits for cold sores, indigestion, genital herpes, high cholesterol, and heartburn. Lemon balm has been used for centuries, even historically being steeped in wine to help lift the spirits. In addition, it can help to heal wounds and treat skin discomfort caused by insect stings or included in a cream to treat cold sores. When combined with valerian or chamomile or hops, it can be a very effective relaxation aid. The easiest application is simply to chop some lemon balm into various cooking dishes like omelets, pork, lamp, soup, fruit salads, and more.

Growing lemon balm at home is relatively easy. The plants should be initially grown indoors and transplanted outside. Plants should be placed in a shady area with partial sunshine. Barely cover the seeds and keep watering to a minimum. Once there are shoots, it can be transplanted into the garden. The soil should be kept moist.

10.   **<u>Marshmallow</u>** (*Althaea officinalis*):

Good for alleviating allergies. The entire plant is edible, so you can toss them into a salad and brew a useful tea. As a perennial herb, marshmallow has been used as a folk remedy to treat colds and cough.

Throat lozenges that contain marshmallow root extract may help cure dry coughs and soothe an irritated throat. In fact, marshmallows that you create a s'more with exist because of this plant. The juice from the marsh mallow plant has been used for centuries as pain relief. In the 1800s, it was mixed with sugar and egg white to be a more pleasant experience for children suffering from a sore throat. It was so popular, that it was marketed as a treat. Marsh mallow is anti-inflammatory and antioxidant so it also relieves symptoms of eczema and dermatitis. An ointment containing 20% marshmallow root extract can help the affected area. This ointment may also act as antibiotic for wounds since the root may have some analgesic properties as well. Currently, there are some studies aimed at discovering the benefit of marshmallow root in repairing the lining of the intestinal tract. If you do take marshmallow root for any ailment, be sure to only take it as a supplement for one month. You then need to take a break before resuming.

Marshmallow is a perennial weed that flowers and is fond of moist, damp places. The leaves have a similar shape with a maple leaf and the flowers, usually white, mauve or pink, have five heart-shaped petals. Its flowers, leaves, and roots are edible.

11.   **Oregano** (*Origanum vulgare*):

It is one of the oldest known herbs used for treating a

variety of conditions. In fact, Hippocrates used it as an antiseptic. It can also be used to treat respiratory tract disorders, urinary track disorders and menstrual cramps. Topically, it can also be used to treat acne and dandruff. This popular herb is one of nature's strongest antibiotics, and some studies show it can be effective against a wide range of food pathogens. In 2014 scientists released information that some popular culinary herbs such as marjoram, oregano, and rosemary may have the potential to help manage diabetes. Lesser known uses of oregano include alleviation of muscle pain, toothaches, heart conditions, cold sores, earache, sore throat, and fatigue.

Oregano is easy to care for and can thrive either in pots or a garden setting. Make sure to put it in a warm, sunny spot with light soil. It can be a good addition to a vegetable garden as it can help to keep pests away that might impact broccoli or beans. The plants have pink flowers and can be terrific ground cover. Be careful where you plant it as it can sometimes go crazy and spread.

12. **<u>Parsley</u>** (*Petroselinum crispum*):

Parsley is a good source of vitamin C, vitamin K, and iron. This can improve skin health, promote faster healing of skin ailments, and strengthen immune and circulatory systems. In fact, some studies show that it has more vitamin C than an orange. Parsley is a natural antioxidant, which can help to reduce bad breath and oral infections. Parsley may help with digestion and flatulence. As it is an antibiotic and antioxidant, it may help to prevent some cancers, and treat osteoporosis and diabetes. Chopped fresh parsley applied to a new bruise may help ease pain and reduce inflammation. A great first-aid secret would be to freeze some in ice cubes to rub on bruises; the parsley helps with the bruise and the ice will reduce inflammation further. Take note that since parsley contains so much vitamin K, people who are taking blood-thinning medicine should watch consumption. Large amounts of parsley may cause uterine contractions, so pregnant women may want to avoid it also.

This biennial herb can be slow to germinate, so you can help to speed up the growth cycle by soaking the seeds in water overnight before planting. Parsley likes rich, slightly damp soil in full sun or partial shade. Parsley self-sows, so be prepared that it may spread when planting in a garden. If you do plant in a garden, good location would be close to corn, asparagus, or tomatoes. If you grow roses, you can plant near those as well. When harvesting, remember that the leaf stems have three segments. Cut leaves from the outer sections of the plant so that the inner portions can replenish and mature. You can harvest the stalks and keep them in a container of water in the refrigerator. Alternately, you can dry the leaves and use them as flavorings.

13.   **<u>Peppermint</u>** (*Mentha x piperita*):

Peppermint is a hybrid of spearmint and water mint that has a wide variety of uses from mouth fresheners, dental products, soothing balms, gum, headache rubs, candies, and more. This may be one of the oldest medicinal herbs used by man. It can easily be grown in a garden where the plants are assured of sufficient water if you give it plenty of room to spread.

Sipping tea made from peppermint leaves can help calm stomach upsets and relieve pain and discomfort due to gas. Carry a few sprigs of peppermint when you travel. If you inhale the aroma of peppermint, it may help prevent nausea and vomiting associated with motion sickness. It's easy to carry a tube of peppermint essential oil when traveling via a plane or in the car if motion sickness begins.

Members of the mint family contain an ingredient called menthol, which is very aromatic and has a cooling effect on the skin. Peppermint oil is a useful ingredient in balms that treat headaches and cold symptoms. It's easy to make a poultice of peppermint leaves that can be applied on the skin which could help relieve the itch and burn from skin allergies and inflammatory conditions. Menthol has slight analgesic action, which is why it is included in balms to help relieve headaches and muscle cramps.

Mint is a perennial plant that thrives in light soil that is moist but with good drainage. Most varieties will put up with shade. If planted outside, the plants spread and will cover the ground rather easily. If planted in a garden, they should be positioned near tomatoes or cabbage. If you are growing in a pot, use compost or fertilizer every few months. Protect the plants or bring indoors during winter and cold climate. Most varieties will tolerate some shade and the variegated types may require some protection from direct sun. For growing outdoors, plant one or two purchased plants (or one or two cuttings from a friend) about 2 feet apart in moist soil. One or two plants will easily cover the ground. Mint should grow to 1 or 2 feet tall.

14. **<u>Plantain</u>** (*Plantago major*)**:**

This may be popularly known as a weed, but it definitely has some medicinal uses. It can cleanse your blood, so it's good for liver health and can draw toxins out of your system. Although not native to North America, it was introduced here by settlers from Europe and Asia and can now be found in local stores. Although the leaves are edible, their flavor might not fit everyone's liking as they are more bitter than spinach.

For heartburn, indigestion, and ulcers, the leaves can also be brewed into a tea or made into a tincture. Adding plantain into an ointment can help with rashes, cuts, bruises, and insect bites. It is also known to help with indigestion, heartburn, and ulcers when taken orally. Since it is a natural antibiotic with anti-inflammatory properties, the ointment will help speed-up the recovery process. The tea or tincture can also be spread or sprayed onto insect bites to help relieve itching. For anyone who suffers from poison sumac, poison ivy, or poison oak, soaking the affected area with plantain tea will ease the suffering. Drops made from plantain can also be used to help with ear infections if the ear drum is still intact (has not burst). These drops will help to shorten the length of the infection and lessen the pain associated with it.

Greater Plantain is a low growing plant and will only reach the height of a foot or so. The plants, with little white flowers, prefers full sun or partial shade.

15.   __Pot Marigold__ (*Calendula officinalis*):

Calendula (aka "Pot Marigold") is one of the most popular edible flowers. Keep in mind that it is not in the same genus as the common marigold. However, they are part of the same family, along with daisies and chrysanthemums. The edible flowers can be used to treat a variety of problems related to the skin like sunburn, acne, blemishes, cuts, bruises, and such. It can help to stop bleeding and reduce inflammation when applied on a wound. A tea made of the steeped flowers is often ingested to get relief from digestive issues and varicose veins. In addition, calendula may help to lower a fever, ease a headache, improve circulation, and block histamines. If you add calendula into your hair rinse, it may help to cover greying hair and ease dry scalp. With great skin healing properties, calendula is a good addition to salves, body products, and soap. As its edible right out of the ground, it is easy to add to salads for simple nutrition. Many people grow pot marigolds because they are bright and cheery and bloom profusely. Most commonly, the blooms are yellow and orange, but there are more subtle colors in cream and pink. Pot marigolds will bloom throughout the growing season.

16.   **<u>Rosemary</u>** (*Rosmarinus officinalis*):

Rosemary is more of a shrub than an herb, but still is an impressive plant for the aroma, the flavor, and the health benefits. Anyone who has ever bought a rosemary tree around Christmas time can attest to the terrific aroma that surrounds the plant. Belonging to the mint family, rosemary is primarily used for general wellbeing, but not for specific diseases.

Some studies indicate rosemary helps to prevent the formation of carcinogens caused by grilling foods. Thus, it's a great addition to grilled chicken, pork, or lamb. It is also known to cleanse and detox the body and fight cirrhosis. Rosemary can be used as an antiseptic and as an ingredient in antibacterial agents.

Recent research in rosemary, specifically the carnosic acid of the plant, indicates that it may improve the brain and address some memory issues. Rosemary oil plays a role in similar studies.

Rosemary can be grown in a pot or planted as an aromatic hedge along a garden. In a garden, they do well around sage, carrots, cabbage, and beans. In a pot, remember that rosemary is a shrub, so it will grow taller than a typical houseplant; make sure that the plant does not become pot-bound. Leaves can easily be harvested and used in cooking and herbal teas. this grows best in hot and dry climates.

17.   **<u>Sage</u>** (*Salvia officinalis*):

Research indicates that sage might improve memory and reduce inflammation. In addition, sage can serve as a natural aid in combating anxiety and nervous disorders, improve appetite, and prevent flatulence. Luckily, it tastes great in a lot of dishes and can easily be incorporated into cooking dishes.

Sage may have a hormone regulatory effect on women. A tea made from the leaves can be used to relieve symptoms of menstrual pain, PMS, and menopause. Asthma might be treated by inhaling an infusion of sage. Alzheimer's, dementia, and depression might be alleviated by sage as well.
Sage is a great herb to use in cooking and is easy to grow, even in small containers in your kitchen. Over-watering is the biggest threat because sage doesn't like wet ground and mildew is a concern. Sage will produce the most flavorful leaves when it receives a lot of sunlight. If planted in an herb garden, it performs well when planted near strawberries, carrots, cabbage, and tomatoes. With slightly alkaline soil and infrequent fertilization, sage will grow a little slower but will provide a more intense flavor.

Containers should be placed in an area with medium to full sun exposure.

18. **<u>St. John's Wort</u>** (*Hypericum perforatum*):

Although popular as an antidepressant, this herb can also help with back pain. It can help to alleviate feelings of sadness, grief, depression, and Seasonal Affective Disorder. But it should be used carefully as it can interact with certain prescription drugs. Luckily, unlike a lot of herbal remedies, there is a lot of scientific studies and information on this particular herb. Your medical doctor might even recommend taking this for minor bouts of depression.

It is typically found in oil, capsule, tincture, or raw form. St. John's wort contains bioflavonoids and antioxidants that can affect chemical and hormonal balances in the body. For the anti-depressant aspects, this herb contains a chemical that may delay or completely inhibit neurotransmitters in the brain such as dopamine, serotonin, and norepinephrine. In this same regard, St. John's wort can also help with anxiety by changing the hormonal balance in the body. This can help with irritability, sleep disturbances, metabolism, and chronic fatigue. By helping to eliminate cortisol and other stress hormones, overall health can improve. As it changes the hormonal balance, it is thought to help women with PMS and menopause symptoms as well, lessening the anxiety and mood swings that can occur.

Further studies are being conducted on the benefits of St. John's wort for those suffering from addiction and withdrawal. Some data has shown that this herb may be helpful for those quitting addictive substances such as alcohol or nicotine. In addition, further studies are being done into the antiviral abilities of this herb as well.

For gardening, St. John's Wort isn't particularly about the soil type and adapts to both dry or moist soil, even if it has to tolerate a drought or soggy conditions occasionally. Plant the herb in a location with a nice balance of shade and sun – too much shade and you won't get enough flowers. When planting, make sure you know that there is a potential for photo-toxicity so grazing animals should be kept away.

19. **Thyme** (*Thymus linearis*):

This lovely smelling herb attracts bees and is a pretty addition to any garden. It spreads easily and is hardy. It has pretty purple flowers. Can be used to treat colds and the flu. With disinfectant properties, it is useful as a gargle for a sore throat. In fact, thyme essential oil is often used as a natural cough remedy. As an alternative, drinking thyme tea may help a sore throat as well.

Thyme is full of vitamin C and is a good source of vitamin A. So, adding thyme to your diet may help boost your immune system and fight off colds.

Essential oil of thyme may be a natural way to fight off mold in your house and can be used as a disinfectant. You can also make a homemade insect repellant out of thyme oil by making a mixture of olive oil and thyme oil in a 1:4 ratio. You can substitute water for the olive oil, but it will not be as structured. In fact, a mixture of thyme oil and olive oil as a moisturizer may boost your mood and increase your positive feelings.

As thyme is frequently used in cooking, you will find this herb in a lot of herb gardens. It can tolerate indirect light, which means it can even be grown inside those little kitchen herb gardens. The pot should have sufficient drainage as thyme doesn't like wet roots. Allow the pot to dry out in between watering. Keep the woody stems cut back to encourage new growth and when the flowers come, trim them and dry for use as a tea. Removing the flowers will only increase production. During the summer, you can set the plants outside to get some extra sunshine and fresh air, but make sure you give it time to acclimate to the different lighting conditions. Trim the stems and remove the leaves by running your fingers down the stem in the opposite direction of growth. Chop leaves and use as seasoning.

20.   **<u>Valerian</u>** (*Valeriana officinalis*):

Lovely and useful. Typically associated with supplements to help you relax and sleep, either in capsule or tea form. It can be used to reduce feelings of anxiety and reduce pain. Precautions on most bottles of Valerian indicate that you should not be taking a daily dose for more than one month at a time. In addition, a variety of other uses have been showing up. Studies indicate that a psychoactive compound present in valerian root may help to reduce or relieve anxiety. This herb may also be useful in reducing the symptoms of ADHD (attention deficit hyperactivity disorder) as it contains the ability to energize a chemical in the brain known as GABA; it may affect OCD symptoms as well. Menopause symptoms may be lessened with the use of valerian as it may help to reduce hot flashes. Valerian may improve your blood flow, strengthening your blood vessel pliability, and improving the heart muscle; and as it is a sedative, it will improve your heart rate. Users of the supplement have indicated that it has helped with Restless Leg Syndrome and studies are being conducted to find out if this is a consistent health benefit.

It is a perennial plant that has white flowers that attract bees and butterflies to your garden. The plant must have full sun exposure for about six (6) hours a day. It likes a well-draining, nitrogen-rich soil but appreciates plenty of moisture. Give the plants plenty of space as they can grow to about five (5) feet high and as much as 12 inches wide. Harvest time is usually the best in spring and fall.

21.   **Yarrow** (*Achillea millefolium*):

Useful in treating wounds, reducing fevers, alleviate allergies, and fight colds. This herb can induce sweating.

This is another ancient herbal treatment possibly dating back to 1000 BC and closely related to another common herbal medicine, chamomile. It boosts the immune system and can soothe cold symptoms. It is considered as an astringent, antiseptic, and anti-inflammatory agent. Tea helps digestion and upset stomach. Topically, the essential oil can reduce eczema related pain, itching, and swelling. Yarrow in boiling water creates a steam that can be inhaled to help clear congestion and control coughing. It is sometimes used as a sedative to help relieve symptoms of insomnia or anxiety. Historically, this herb was consumed like a vegetable and was eaten and prepared like spinach. As a seasoning, it can be used as an alternative to tarragon because the flavor is similar. In powdered form, yarrow can be spread onto a wound to help stop bleeding and lessen pain. Since it's a natural antiseptic, it will keep the wound from getting infected. A poultice made from yarrow has been known to help breast-feeding women who are suffering from mastitis, providing quick relieve for the pain of cracked nipples. Yarrow may have some digestive benefits by lessening cramps, flatulence, or diarrhea by reducing muscle spasms along the GI tract. It also has cardiovascular benefits because it helps to lower blood pressure and improve the respiratory system, alleviating asthma symptoms.

Yarrow is versatile and hardy perennial. It has showy flower heads that are made up of a bunch of tiny, tightly-packed flowers. These flowers may be pink, red, yellow, or a number of shades in between. It is a nice addition to the garden, as it attracts butterflies, smells nice, and is drought-resistant.

The herb should be planted in the spring because it likes hot and dry conditions. Make sure that the soil is well-drained. Soil should be average because if it is too rich, your growth will take over and you'll be required to trim it regularly. Put the plants about 12-24 inches apart as they will spread and grow to about four (4) feet tall. In the spring, a thin layer of compost will help them grow.

Chapter 3: Beneficial Herbs to Add to Your Medicine Chest

Herb	Description of Benefits
abscess root	May reduce fever, treat cough or reduce inflammation.
agrimony	Improves vision, can help to heal wounds, ease digestive issues, treat cough and sore throat, or as a sleep aid. Primarily used as a tea.
alder buckthorn	Used as a laxative; dangerous in large doses.
aniseed	Digestive aid (reduces gas and eases nausea) and increases milk supply in breastfeeding women. Can help to alleviate anxiety and ease cold symptoms.
arnica	Anti-inflammatory. It should not be taken internally but is beneficial as an ointment for reducing the appearance of bruises and mild muscle pain.
asafetida	May be useful in treating breathing problems, IBS or high cholesterol.
ashwagandha	Best-known to boost sexual drive and fertility. Also known to enhance memory, boost energy, and help to alleviate stress and anxiety.

Herb	Description of Benefits
aspalathus	Antioxidant similar to bilberry. Boosts eye health and immune function.
astragalus	Strengthens the immune system.
Avaram Senna	Has laxative properties, eases conjunctivitis, treats diabetes, and alleviates urinary tract issues.
balloon flower	Anti-microbial, anti-inflammatory, relieves allergies, improves insulin levels, lowers cholesterol.
belladonna	Although toxic, this has been used by women to enlarge their pupils to enhance beauty (the translation is "beautiful woman"). Can be included in small dosages as a sedative.
bilberry	A powerful antioxidant that is relatively unknown. It has positive effects on the brain and heart. Protects the retina and improves vision.
bilwa	Used in India to help treat eye conditions (sties and conjunctivitis).
bitter orange	Alleviates nausea, constipation, and indigestion.
bitter melon	Helps reduce blood glucose levels.

Herb	Description of Benefits
black cohosh	Anti-inflammatory and rejuvenating herb with immune-boosting properties. Popular in supplements for women to combat menstrual and menopausal complications. Also believed to improve good circulation, help lower blood pressure, and improve heart health. Should not be used by pregnant or nursing women.
black walnut	This herb has been used as an anti-parasitic, anti-fungal, digestive aid, and cure poison ivy, and treatment for warts.
blue snakeweed	May ease malaria symptoms; treats dysentery, livery disorders, may control diabetes; anti-inflammatory properties.
borage	Used to alleviate colic, cramps, diarrhea, urinary tract disorders.
burdock	Used as a diuretic; lowers blood sugar and eases symptoms of the common cold.
cardamom	Anti-microbial properties. Can rid the blood of bad cholesterol and improve circulation. May serve as an anti-depressant, anti-inflammatory, and anti-spasmodic. Can improve the health and function of male sexual organs.

Herb	Description of Benefits
catnip	Can be a digestive aid (reduces gas). The tea can relieve cold symptoms and reduce fever by inducing sweating. When applied to wounds, it can help stop bleeding and reduce swelling. Easy to grow and produces beautiful purple flowers.
charcoal tree	May be used to treat a sore throat, toothaches, bronchitis, asthma, and gonorrhea. And may be beneficial as a general antidote to general poisoning.
chasteberry	Used for hundreds of years to control female hormone imbalances (combatting PMS, breast tenderness, hot flashes, mood swings, and boosting milk production in lactating mothers).
chickweed	Relieves itchy skin, remedy for pulmonary diseases, may help with anemia, bronchitis, RA and menstrual pain.
cinnamon	Can be used to treat minor wounds as an anti-bacterial agent and can be an ingredient in anti-viral topical treatments and oral remedies.
cinquefoil	Reduces inflammation, helps to alleviate jaundice, treats ulcers and mouth sores.

Herb	Description of Benefits
clove bud	Enhances the immune system as it is an antioxidant, anti-bacterial and anti-microbial agent. May treat toothaches.
comfrey	Reduces inflammation and relieves digestive issues.
common nettle	Treat kidney and UT disorders, symptoms of gout, and the flu.
coriander	The seeds help to balance blood sugar by stimulating the pancreas to produce insulin. Coriander can also help liver function and improves cholesterol levels. It is a natural antibiotic, so it could help in the treatment of food-borne pathogens (such as salmonella). Good source of fiber, vitamins A and K, antioxidants, potassium, iron, and magnesium.
cranberry	Anyone who has ever had a bladder infection can use cranberry supplements but can also be used to fight prostatitis.
cypress	Antiseptic and astringent. The prime ingredient in natural sedatives and respiratory mixtures. Also used as a diuretic.
daisy	Treats disorders of the respiratory or GI tract.
dill	Ease upset stomach, help to alleviate insomnia, may treat colic.

Herb	Description of Benefits
elderberry	Historically, the flowers have been used in flu remedies and antiviral mixes (topical and oral). Can treat pain, reduce swelling, alleviate coughs, fevers, constipation, and sinus infections.
eucalyptus	Antiviral, antibacterial, and anti-infectious properties. This herb is a well-known component of a lot of cold remedies.
evening primrose	The oil used as an anti-inflammatory and can help with eczema.
fenugreek	May help with diabetes, menopause, and digestive ailments.
garden angelic	Alleviate disorders of the GI tract, fevers, infections, and symptoms of the flu.
geranium	Can detoxify the liver and stop the bleeding of wounds. It is also an antibacterial and anti-infectious agent.
ginkgo biloba	Improves blood flow to the eyes (helps with macular degeneration). May help ears by preventing tinnitus, inner ear disturbances, and other conditions. Can help with asthma, bronchitis, fatigue, or Alzheimer's.

Herb	Description of Benefits
ginseng	Relieves and prevents fatigue (mental and physical). Reduces the severity and frequency of colds. Possibly beneficial to those suffering from erectile dysfunction.
goldenrod	Treats painful menstrual cramps; externally can be applied to eczema and skin ulcers.
goldenseal	Reduces the inflammation associated with conjunctivitis and sties.
greenthread	(aka Navajo tea) A diuretic, anti-inflammatory, natural remedy for urinary tract infections, and sooths gastrointestinal distress.
hepatica (common)	Treats liver disease; eases bronchitis and gout.
hibiscus	Boosts fluid balance in the body, maintains normal body temperature, and enhances heart health.
hollyhock (common)	Used as a laxative and controls inflammation
hops	Associated with beer-making, hops can also be used to induce sleep, alleviate stress, and lessen menopause issues (hot flashes and others).
horse chestnut	Extract from the seed can be used to treat varicose veins, reduce swelling in the feet and legs.

Herb	Description of Benefits
horsetail	Heals ulcers, treat wounds, kidney problems, and can help to stop bleeding.
hyssop	An anti-microbial agent that treats respiratory infections and skin conditions. Fights fungal infections, the flu, and strep. This herb has been around a long time and is one of the oldest known medicinal herbs. Closely related to marjoram and oregano.
Indian sandalwood	Treats urinary tract infections, common cold, bronchitis, fever, and gallbladder disorders.
karvy	Anti-microbial, anti-inflammatory (may help with RA)
kava	Relieves anxiety with significant muscle-relaxing effects. May also be used to treat urinary tract infections or asthma.
kratom	Has gained popularity recently as an aid to relieve withdrawal symptoms for people suffering from addiction.
licorice	Treat sore throats and cough, calms gastrointestinal tract issues.

Herb	Description of Benefits
lovage	Serves as a digestive aid (reduces gas), eases a sore throat, eases pain from stomach ulcers. Can be added to a bath to ease pain and inflammation resulting from skin conditions. Belongs to the carrot family.
Mahonia grape extract	Reduces the impact of sun damage on the eyes while helping to strengthen the retina, can slow eye aging and improve overall eye health.
marjoram	Possesses antibacterial and anti-infectious properties. May soothe sore muscles and regulate blood pressure.
milk thistle	Remedy for kidney problems. Can be used to alleviate the harmful effects of exposure to environmental toxins and alcohol poisoning.
myrrh	One of the oldest known herbs and was mentioned in the Christian Bible. Can soothe skin rashes, impair nerve spasms, and boost the immune system. An anti-infectious and antiviral agent.
neem	Used to treat worms, skin infections, malaria, and RA.
noni	May relieve joint pain and skin conditions.

Herb	Description of Benefits
passionflower	Assists with vision issues. Helps to alleviate eye strain if you spend all day staring at a screen. Relaxes the small blood vessels in the eye. Thought to have some anti-depressant properties.
pennyroyal	Eases headaches and colic lessens feverish symptoms
poppy	Soothes coughs, promotes sleep, eases asthma and whooping cough
primrose	Promotes sleep, reduces tension, eases headaches, and treats gout.
purslane	Anti-bacterial and anti-fungal properties.
red clover	Detoxifies the blood and body. The tea can be an effective treatment for cold symptoms.
rosewood	Fights infections, both bacterial and viral.
slippery elm	Approved by the FDA to treat minor throat irritations and a cough resulting from a cold or heartburn.
spearmint	Aids in treating bronchial problems and nervous system issues.
summer savory	Anti-bacterial and anti-fungal uses.

Herb	Description of Benefits
sweet cicely	Known as Spanish Chervil and Garden Myrrh. Can be used as a natural sweetener. It may also treat anxiety and hypertension, ease digestive problems, and detoxify the urinary tract.
sweet marjoram	High in beneficial nutrients such as vitamins A, C, K, iron, potassium, calcium, zinc, magnesium, and manganese. Anti-microbial and aids with digestion.
sweet violet	Alleviates cold and flu symptoms. Serves as a pain reliever for headaches and muscle soreness. Can help detoxify (diuretic). Relaxant and sleep aid.
tarragon	Treats toothaches, may induce menstruation, and eliminate parasites in the intestines.
tea tree	Has an antibiotic property that treats oral and skin issues. Possibly in the top 10 most frequently used herbs as it is added to cosmetic applications as well (shampoo, conditioner, lotions, etc.)
turmeric	Digestive aid, improves liver function and relieves pain associated with arthritis.
verbena	Treat respiratory tract diseases and sore throats.
veronica	Treats sinus and ear infections.

Herb	Description of Benefits
watercress	Diuretic and anti-bacterial.
water germander	Eases symptoms from asthma, fever, hemorrhoids, intestinal parasites, and diarrhea.
white buttercup	Ailments for GI and respiratory diseases and may inhibit fungal activity.
white willow	The precursor of aspirin as a source of salicylic acid.
yellow lady's slipper	Remedy for anxiety, headaches, toothache, and can be used as a sedative.

Chapter 4: How to Prepare Herbs

The time and method of harvesting greatly depends on the type of herb you are harvesting. Some medicinal supplements are sourced from the flowers, some on the seeds, and some on the roots – and some on any and all parts of the plant. Generally, the leaves should be harvested before flowers form. After flowering, a lot of herbs become bitter or their flavors are greatly diminished. When the leaves are harvested, it is actually the oil in the leaves which provides both the fragrance and flavor. Ideally, the leaves should be picked early in the morning before temperatures rise. The leaves should not be washed as that will rinse away the useful oils in the herbs.

For the flowers, some herbs like chamomile and lavender are best when harvested before the flowers fully blooms. When harvesting for seeds, herbs such as coriander, fennel, and caraway need to be harvested just as the pods begin changing colors. For herbs where the roots are most useful, most of those need to be harvested at the end of summer or early autumn. Harvesting annuals can be ongoing and can be done right until frost occurs. However, for perennials, trimming should not occur any later than the dog days of summer as this may encourage new growth that will continue after the season and cold weather that can damage the plant. It pays to know your plants as certain flowering herbs such as tarragon or lavender should be cut back to half their height in early July in order to promote a second bloom in autumn.

Herbs Preservation

Typically, herbs are best used when fresh, especially when cooking. After an herb is picked, the aroma and flavor fade quickly. Once harvested, there are a number of ways to store and preserve herbs for future use. A lot of herbs like parsley, basil, cilantro, and basil can be stored on the kitchen counter in a glass of water. Just like an arrangement of fresh flowers. Trim the ends of the stems and give them an inch or two of water to feed them. Those types of herbs will remain fresh for about a week in this fashion. For others, such as chives, thyme, and rosemary, they are best stored in a refrigerator. Herbs should be wrapped in a damp towel and stored in the refrigerator. There are also a number of storage containers available on the market that can help to prolong the life of fresh herbs. None of the herbs should be rinsed off before they are stored because this will diminish their flavor and hasten wilting. In addition, the longer herbs are stored, the less their potency will be.

Drying your herbs will allow you the longest storage length and will retain the highest quality and flavor. Stored properly, dried herbs can be flavorful and helpful for 24-36 months but are most potent within 12 months. For long term storage, and to retain the highest flavor and quality, consider drying herbs.

Dried herbs can be kept for two or three years but should really be used within a year. Any storage time longer than this, will cause the decline of taste and aroma. Sun, oven, or dehydrator drying is not recommended, because the herbs will lose too much flavor and color.

When using an oven, the temperature should be set between 180 and 200 degrees only. Keep the door open in order to let moisture escape. You must watch the herbs closely and repeatedly stir the layer of herbs to ensure they dry completely and do not burn. For a dehydrator, a machine will quickly work on drying the herbs – although the racks may need to be rotated to ensure all of the batches are dried evenly. The sun can dry herbs as well but it will need a little longer drying time and a structure may have to be build that will help to ensure that the herbs don't blow away and remain bug-free. Air-drying is another method. Gather the herbs by the stems and hang them upside-down in a warm area (at least 70 degrees F). Make sure the area is not in direct sunlight, but the herbs will take about three (3) weeks to be ready. Be aware that you can minimize the mess this method makes by placing a paper bag over any herbs with seed heads as the seeds will drop into the bag as they dry instead of on the floor. This method will take further processing once the herbs are dried, the leaves will need to be removed and crushed or ground into powder just before use. Some people who use this method frequently will take a picture frame and cover it with netting or screen and use those to hold the herbs while drying. Leaves should be striped and laid in a single-layer on the screen, turning the frame every day. Microwave ovens can also be used for drying. Once the herbs are cleaned, they should be laid in a single-layer on a paper towel and heated in 30 second bursts until they are dry. Great care should be taken and the herbs should not be set on fire. Regardless of which method you use, once herbs are dried and prepared, they should be stored in an airtight container, preferably ceramic or glass. Keep the container away from heat or light. A lot of people keep spices near the stove for the convenience of cooking, but that quickly lessens flavor and fragrance. If possible, keep the leaves whole and crush it just before consumption.

Freezing herbs are another method to preserve herbs for future use. Unlike drying, these herbs should be washed before processing. Once dry, they should be spread into a single layer and placed in the freezer. Once frozen, they can be combined into a container and placed back into the freezer until ready for use. Some herbs freeze better than others and some research should be done to ensure it is the correct approach. Sage, tarragon, dill, basil, chives, thyme, mint, and others will freeze well and remain viable for up to six months. As an alternative approach, you can try painting the leaves with oil, then freeze them. Afterwards, take them out and chop them in a food processor with a little oil to form a paste. The paste can then be frozen either in a block or in small segments (such as a tablespoon or ice-cube tray) so that when cooking, you can easily remove some of the paste and add to soups or stews. If you don't want to add the oil, you can simply add chopped herbs to water and freeze in smaller sections.

Herbal salts can be created by combining salt and spices. Using a glass jar with a lid, simply layer the leaves of the herb with layers of salt, pressing firmly between layers until the jar is full. Seal tightly. Or combine 1 cup of salt with six (6) tablespoons of an herb in a food processor and process until combined. This herbal salt can be stored in an air-tight container. The flavor will be most viable for the first year and will diminish after that.

<u>Harvesting and Growth</u>

As a general rule, when harvesting, you should never take more than a third of the entire growth. This will allow enough of the plant material to remain so that effective regrowth can occur. Although this rule may apply in most cases, some plants are exceptions. For example, chives will grow back faster if they are cut down to less than an inch of exposure from the ground. Other species flourish if they are harvested all at once. Some harvests are based on the time of year, some are based on the size of the plant, some are based on the coloring of the leaves, and others are based on when blooms appear.

Each plant has its own preferred method of harvesting. Annuals that are leafy, like basil, should be harvested by pinching bunches of leaves off the stems from the tips. They should be clipped close to encourage regrowth and more prolific plants. Any herbs that have a longer stem like rosemary, parsley, and lavender, should be cut down next to the base, less than an inch from the ground cover. Perennial herbs that are leafy, like tarragon, sage, oregano, and thyme, can be picked by the stem.

Some plants are harvested to use more than one part – the leaves, the seeds or the roots. For some of those herbs, timing can be everything. Cilantro's leaves are the part of the plant that is being used so it should be harvested before blooming. If you are after coriander, it involves waiting for that same plant to bloom and produce seeds. Those seeds are then harvested to become coriander. Herbs that are based on the flower should be harvested just before the blooms fully open so that they are most potent.

To produce more leaves on herbs like dill or basil requires removal of the flower stalks once they appear. Herbs that bloom, like mint, thyme or oregano, are at their most flavorful just before they begin to bloom, so that is the best time to harvest their leaves.

Herbs can either be grown from seeds or harvested to be grown from the clippings; stalks should be placed in water until they grow roots and then can be transplanted into pots or directly into the garden.

Multiple Uses

Oil and Butter: Combining herbs with butter or olive oil can not only serve to preserve the herbs, it can also be a great addition to cooking. This mixture will cut down on the herbs discoloring or wilting. To ensure the safest preparation method, the herbs must not have any water at the time the mixture is made. If the herbs have any water, it will increase the risk of bacterial contamination.

Vinegars: Herbs can also be preserved by creating flavored vinegar. Mild vinegars work best, like white, rice or white wine. However, for stronger flavored herbs like basil or rosemary, apple cider vinegar can be used for a new flavor combination. Put fresh herbs into containers of vinegar, add a lid, and simply wait until infusion.

Chapter 5: Conclusion

When deciding which herbs to grow, there are multiple factors that should come into play. First is the climate in the area you live in and your gardening abilities. There is nothing more frustrating than trying to grow something that just won't sprout. Then, how much time do you want to devote to the growing, harvesting, and preparation of the herbs? Do you want to get involved in drying and mixing tinctures? Finally, what medicinal conditions do you want to treat – if you suffer from back pain, then maybe you want to focus on those herbs that are helpful in treating inflammation.

As with anything else, it pays to do your research and be informed. The medical condition may be something serious enough to warrant any attempt to cure it. Herbal supplements cover a wide variety of treatments for conditions such a migraine, cold, high blood pressure, and more. Unfortunately, there isn't a lot of reliable scientific studies that have reliably been conducted on how effective herbs can be used as medicine and what the side effects might be. While most manufacturers of herbal supplements meet consistent quality standards, it pays to be informed as to what brands are of high quality because those companies do not need to get approval from the Food and Drug Administration (FDA) before marketing their products. In fact, even when the FDA gets involved, herbal supplements fall under the category of dietary supplements which gives them a different set of rules from food or drug approval. Companies are not allowed to make a scientific or medical claim and must put a disclaimer about any evaluation of any claims for treating conditions.

Notwithstanding regulations and quality concerns, herbal supplements can have powerful effects on the body. Some can interact with prescription medications currently being uses. And some can be more harmful than beneficial when taken in the wrong dosages. Medications such as blood pressure medications or blood thinners may interact with a variety of herbal supplements. If you are currently breast-feeding or pregnant, you should definitely do your research and speak with your physician about any supplements and side effects. If you're having surgery, it is essential that you tell your doctor what herbal medicine you're taking to ensure that your surgeons have all the information necessary to ensure your safety.

When starting a new supplement, do your research and find out the side effects. Begin by taking the lowest recommended dosage and keep track of what your taking and any affects you may be feeling. Choose a brand that has been tested by reputable independent sources and laboratories. Check for any advisors which would indicate adverse effects of the supplement; the FDA website typically contains updates.

Thanks for making it through to the end of

Herbal Apothecary, let's hope it was informative and was able to provide you with all of the tools you need to achieve your goals whatever they may be.

Finally, if you found this book useful in any way, a review on Amazon is always appreciated!

This book belongs to a series of books about herbal medicine and how to use it to improve our life. For more information, visit

www.db-publishing.com

Herbal Medicine Guide for Beginners

All you need to know about how to use Medicinal Herbs and Natural Remedies for Self Healing

Table of Contents

There are no scenarios in which the publisher or the original author of this work can be in any fashion deemed liable for any hardship or damages that may befall them after undertaking information described herein.

Additionally, the information in the following pages is intended only for informational purposes and should thus be thought of as universal. As befitting its nature, it is presented without assurance regarding its prolonged validity or interim quality. Trademarks that are mentioned are done without written consent and can in no way be considered an endorsement from the trademark holder.

Introduction

Congratulations on downloading Herbal Medicine Guide for Beginners and thank you for doing so.

The following chapters will discuss a basic overview of the history of medicinal herbs, from the first man to when herbal medicines became a trading commodity of the world. You will learn the definitions for all of the forms that medicinal herbs can take, what is in the label, and what to look for on the shelf.

There are three chapters providing you with choices of medicinal herbs to treat ailments physically, mentally, and emotionally. Also, we will bring you back to where early man started, being in-charge of your health through the creation of your own medicinal herb garden.

All of the information contained within is practical advice, easy to follow, and designed for your well-being. We encourage you to make medicinal herbs part of your medicine chest and hopefully, part of your everyday health regime. Safer than pharmaceutical options for many of the more common afflictions, medicinal herbs may be the best investment you can make for your future. This guide will lead you into a better quality of life through a deeper appreciation for the world of medicinal herbs.

There are plenty of books on this subject on the market, thanks again for choosing this one! Every effort was made to ensure it is full of as much useful information as possible, please enjoy!

Chapter 1: A Brief History of Medicinal Plants & Herbs

The English Oxford defines a medicinal plant: *(of a substance or plant) having healing properties.*

Today, a medicinal plant is recognized as one which is used for the maintenance of health and/or to be taken to alleviate a specific ailment. This recognition takes place both in modern and traditional forms of medicine. It was conservatively estimated that there are over 17,810 species of plants which have a use for medicinal purposes out of the 30,000 plants documented for possessing a use of any kind. (The Royal Botanic Gardens, Kew, 2016)

Plants, many of which we recognize today as culinary herbs and spices, have been considered since pre-historic times as containing medicinal value. Humans originated with a close connection to their immediate environment, using what was available to them for food and medicine. Flowering plants are the original source of most medicines. These tended to grow near human settlements, such as chickweed, yarrow, dandelion, and nettles. The trial and error approach was taken when these early 'scientists' applied these sources as potential plants to meet their needs. The knowledge gained was transferred from each generation through oral and written traditions, depending on the culture involved. This knowledge has been gradually becoming more complete as civilizations formed and the sharing of knowledge occurs.

Not only do humans use their environment as a source of medicine, animals including primates, sheep, and monarch butterflies, also consume certain medicinal plants when ill.

The earliest evidence known for the use of plants as medicine comes from prehistoric burial sites. Dating back to the Paleolithic period, a 60,000-year-old Neanderthal site in Iraq contained quantities of pollen from eight plant species, seven of which we use today as remedies.

The earliest written evidence comes from clay tablets dating back to the Sumerian civilization. Recorded on them are hundreds of plants, including opium, used for their medicinal values. Papyrus scrolls from ancient Egypt offer details of eight hundred and fifty plant-based medicines. The source of pharmacopeias, *De materia medica*, documented more than 1,000 medicine recipes based on over six hundred different plant sources. This sourcebook was used for over 1,500 years as a reliable resource for medicinal products.

Before 500 B.C., belief systems at that time ascribed both magical and healing properties to plants. Beginning with the age of Hippocrates, after 500 B.C., physical illness was seen as part of the natural human condition and plants began to lose their mythical properties.

Before the 16th century, there are three widely recognized ancient medicinal systems namely the Chinese medicine, European, and Ayurvedic (Indian). All three are based on very different approaches to the human body but all are in agreement with one essential concept. If the body is out of balance, then illness will result. The restoration of balance is required for good health to be present. One should work with nature and the body's own healing capacity complemented by healing herbs to restore balance.

As part of this shared belief system, all three medical practices held, at their core, a belief that each human contains a primal (vital) energy source. This source sustains the health and life and each individual has it to varying degrees. The Chinese defined this source as "qi" and the Ayurvedic's referred to it as "prana". Westerners referred to it simply as the "vital force".

When world trade exploded in the 14th century, the exchange of remedies and herbs between Muslims, the Chinese, Indians, and Europeans increased. Europeans now add access to new herbs and their healing properties, such as ginger, cinnamon, and cardamom. The Far East was introduced to sage and its potential health benefits at the same time.

Unfortunately, European medicine was not able to treat the many plagues and epidemics that swept through the continent during the 12th and 18th centuries. One common modern day interpretation of the Black plague nursery rhyme *Ring around the Rosie* is that people at the time believed you contracted the disease from breathing 'bad air'. So carrying a posy (sachet) of flowers in your pocket would sweeten the air around you, thus ensuring the carrier would not breathe in any disease.

Herbs brought to Europe from Central and South America, thanks to the Spanish and Portuguese explorers, were potent remedies for successfully treating smallpox, syphilis, and malaria. There followed a surge in popularity for homeopathy and herbal medicines.

In the 19th century, the modern medicine took over, dismissing all previously held concepts of herbal medicine as ignorance and superstition. This was the dawning of the age of western medicine and more traditional practices were overshadowed all over the world.

When the British moved in to colonize India, they declare that the practice of Ayurveda was inferior to western medicine and subsequently tried to squash and replace this traditional form.

China, through the maintenance of closing themselves off the Western world, was more successful at maintaining their traditional medical practices. In many western countries, it became illegal to practice herbal medicine without receiving an official qualification.

People continue to access the healing powers of many plants and herbs, visiting naturopaths, shamans, homeopaths, herbologists, etc. In 1991, the World Health Organization (WHO) formulated a policy on the use of traditional medicines. They have since then published guidelines on the more widely used ones. WHO has estimated, due to a lack of reliable data, up to 80% of our current world population relies on traditional medicine, with approximately two billion of these mainly reliant on medicinal plants. One reason for this is the affordability of plant-based medicines making them more accessible to many people.

In developed countries, there is an increase in the use of plant-sourced medicines which include health care or herbal care products. The benefits from these sources are not always scientifically known as there has been no means of testing the pharmaceutical benefits of each dosage. Since the medicinal value of each plant is dependent on many variables like the soil, sun, a strain of plant, and time of harvesting, it is difficult to assess the benefits and toxicity of these remedies. Although many of these herbal remedies have been in use since early man, there is still very little knowledge of the pharmacological base for their status as a medicinal plant.

Current drug research does make use of ethnobotany to look for active medicinal substances in plants. This research has produced the discovery of hundreds of compounds which are all useful to the medical industry. The most common ones we know of are aspirin (willow bark), quinine, (Remijia bark or Cinchona bark), opium (dried latex from the opium poppy), and digoxin (foxglove flower).

Over a quarter of modern drugs prescribed to patients are sourced from medicinal plants and are rigorously tested prior to use. In some non-industrialized countries, medicinal plants can make up the majority of treatments without the same scientific research. Although there is still little regulation, WHO still does coordinate a network for the safe and practical use of such plants.

Today, there is an annually global export market value of several hundred billion USD in 2017. This market is made up of up to 70,000 plants with anticipated medicinal values. Given that there is little regulation worldwide in the market, medicinal plants face the threat of over-collection to meet demands. Furthermore, climate change and on-going habitat destruction are affecting the viability of these potent medicinal sources. By actively engaging in a deeper awareness of traditional medical knowledge, we can play a key role in a sustained exploitation of these natural resources.

In almost every culture in the world, plants are used as a medical resource. In industrialized nations, the efficacy, safety, and quality of these plants (herbal drugs) have very recently become a key issue. Through the standardization and evaluation of the active plant-derived medical compounds, medicinal plants can assist as an emerging boon to our current healthcare system. Herbal drugs could be the stimulus for future cures of many human diseases. Collaboration with different cultures on their medicinal plant practices is required for the creation of historically accurate accounts for the benefit of the people all over the world.

Beyond their medicinal value, medicinal plants have the potential to increase the quality of life through socio-economic benefits. There is the financial benefit to those who cultivate them for sale, in addition to job opportunities, income via taxation, and a healthier labor force worldwide. The market should be encouraged and further developed through improved practices in the processing and distribution, further scientific research into their medicinal value, and improved financing for those trying to cultivate them.

In the United States most herb product manufacturers already have their products sourced through domestic and foreign markets. The medicinal herb manufacturing industry has been in a steady growth for a number of years and it has matured. Note the number of products readily available in grocery stores, pharmacies, even dollar stores. Probably the best method of purchasing choice organically grown medicinal herb products is by buying products made from from small local manufacturers. Because these companies do not buy in the amounts internationals do they will be the ones purchasing from the local farmer closest to them. By supporting local business you are encouraging diversity and sustainability in the medicinal herb products market.

Chapter 2: What to Look For In Your Modern Day Medicinal Herbs and Where to Find Them

In this chapter, we will use herb and plant interchangeably with the understanding that an herb is the whole or part of a whole plant which, for the definition of this Guide, is used for its medicinal properties.

Herbal products are defined as being formulated from plants to treat diseases and maintain health. These can come in the form of gels, lotions, salves, ointments, and creams which can be applied directly to your skin. Some products are water soluble and are used in the bath.

There are also essences where the volatile oil of the herb is extracted through a steam distillation. The resulting oil can then be added to your bath, inhaled as a scent, or rubbed on the skin. Some oil like that of oregano is even ingested internally defining this one as a supplement rather than a product.

Poultices and plasters, which involve a soft collection of plant material, are laid on the afflicted body part to relieve the swelling and inflammation. This mass is typically held in place with a cloth.

Herbal supplements are products made from plants and designed only for internal use. These can contain parts of or the whole plant itself. Herbal supplements are sold as pills, tablets, powders, extracts, tinctures, teas, dried, and fresh cuttings of the plant itself.

Pills are used as a general term to define either a capsule or a tablet. They are round and oval, whereas a tablet is flat and circular.

A tablet, which is made up of compressed powder in a solid form, is designed to be cut into two parts.

Capsules contain either a powder or a jelly in a dissolvable gel container. The contents of the capsules are dissolved into the bloodstream immediately.

Teas, also known as infusions, are created by soaking the fresh or dried herbs in hot water and letting them seep. These can then be drunk cold or hot.

A decoction is created by simmering the bark,

roots, or berries in hot water for long periods of time. These can also be consumed hot or cold.

Tinctures are created through the soaking of an herb in an alcohol and water solution. This process concentrates and preserves the active ingredients in the herb. Tinctures can vary in their strength and are expressed through a ratio of the weight of the dried herb to the volume of the finished product. Extracts involve soaking the plant in a solvent which removes certain types of chemicals. The resulting liquid can be used as is or evaporated to create a dry powder for use in tablets or capsules.

In 1994, in the United States, the Dietary Supplement Health and Education Act became law. As defined by Congress, a supplement for safe use is one which:

- is used with the intention of supplementing the diet.

- contains one or more of the following as ingredients – herbs, botanicals, amino acids, vitamins, minerals, and other substances,

- the intention is to ingest this orally as a liquid, pill, tablet, capsule, tea, or tincture,

- is clearly and accurately labeled on the front of the bottle as a supplement.

Herbal supplements can range in effect from a mild action with very subtle effects noted over a long period of time to very potent results. Many of the liquid supplements have varying strengths, dependent on if it is a tea, a tincture, or even an extract. A difference in how the supplement is prepared and the concentration of the chemical recovered from the plant can affect the outcome of how it is used. For example, peppermint tea is a fairly mild digestive aid but peppermint oil is very concentrated and can be toxic if not taken correctly. It is important to read the labeling on the supplement or, if you are using the whole herb, consult with a professional for an accurate dosage.

Since the FDA does not consider herbal supplements as drugs (they are classified as food under the Act), they are not subject to the same testing and regulatory standards as drugs. On the labels, the supplements list how the herbs can influence different physical responses but they are not allowed to say they can treat specific conditions.

Determining a manufacturer's claims of quality can depend on hearsay, a doctor's opinion, or even the label itself. Since 2007, there has been something called the Good Manufacturing

Process for dietary supplements. These are a list of requirements and expectations which manufacturers have to adhere to for the identification, concentration, purity, and quality of their product. This is in an attempt to prevent the wrongful inclusion of contaminated ingredients, an imbalance of ingredients, and the improper labeling of their product.

We have talked about what to look for when purchasing packaged and prepared medicinal herbs. You can locate these alternatives at health food stores, dietary supplement stores, pharmacies, and even in your big chain grocery stores. While these options are a great alternative to chemicals, there is always the option of creating your own remedies at home. This option will be discussed further in Chapter Six, Growing Your Own Medicinal herbs.

If you do not have the option to garden and want to go pick some herbs, here are a few practical tips to follow.

Rule One. Identify what you are picking correctly. It is extremely easy to confuse some herbs which are indistinguishable in looks but contain very different properties for healing purposes.

Rule Two. Always pick more than a mile off the highway. There are some herbs that seem to thrive on car exhaust fumes. Plants picked next to a busy road may have up to 200 times their natural lead content.

Rule Three. If your herb of choice is growing profusely in a given area, this is a good indication that the soil is nutrient and mineral-rich which is promoting that healthy growth. Picking your herbs from areas such as these is a good choice.

Rule Four. Pick your herbs once the dew has evaporated from the leaves, around mid-morning. Many plants will develop mold after picking if there is any dampness on them.

Rule Five. Select only the best plants, avoiding the ones that display any signs of disease or damage. Drooping leaves, black spots or a discolored stem are all signs that the plant is not a healthy one.

A great advantage to using medicinal herbs as a therapy or health enhancement is that it is totally safe especially when it is administered correctly. Beware of the publicity that erroneously states that medicinal herbs can be swallowed in random amounts without any ill effects occurring. Not only is this incorrect, it is also very dangerous.

Medicinal herbs are safer than current western medications but they still must be taken with the awareness of accurate dosage. Always check with a professional what the correct dosage of medicinal herbs you should be taking. Certain plants used for benign purposes are extremely toxic and can create very harmful side effects if not taken with care. Unless you have the medical certification qualifying you to prescribe medication, do not treat anything more than a minor illness at home. Always talk to professionals about any serious health concerns. If your minor illness is not responding to your medicinal herbal remedies, you should seek professional advice. Keep in mind that if you have any doubts regarding a medicinal herb best not to take it until you can confer with an expert in herbal medicines.

Chapter 3:   External Physical Uses and the Specific Herbs

This chapter will cover six of the more common ailments that can afflict the average human. Although the frequency of these may vary with our age and our physical activity level, most of us will experience at least two of these ailments at least one time in our life.

Cuts and Bruises

Probably the number one cross-generational ailment there is. It is also one of the ones that we can be assured will go away with time.

Arnica is top of the list for its medicinal power. Used for centuries, this pretty plant can be applied topically (cream, essential oil or tincture) for treating bruises and offering some pain relief right at the source. Arnica can also be taken orally as a form of homeopathy, providing healing for physical and emotional trauma.

Comfrey is well respected in permaculture gardens as it reproduces like crazy while improving the soil at the same time. For humans, Comfrey is respected for its active ingredient, allantoin which is a compound that assists with increasing the speed of cellular growth which is extremely beneficial with the healing of cuts, bruises, and even broken bones. Comfrey is normally applied in poultice form.

Chamomile is not only a yummy cup of tea. It is also an anti-inflammatory with antibacterial properties. Wet tea bags can be applied directly to cuts for the best treatment results.

Eucalyptus is known for its consumption by koala bears and the medicinal smell of its leaves. This smell is redolent of the antiseptic properties contained in those leaves making it a good poultice for pain reduction in muscle and joint injuries or used as an ointment for small cuts. If using Eucalyptus in oil form, be sure to dilute it before applying to the affected area.

Plantain can be found all over your yard. You can easily find one if you have been bitten by a bee or spider. Chew a few leaves to get the juices flowing then apply directly to the bitten area, barring that you can find it in a tincture or salve form. Plantain is also useful for bruises and cuts.

Tea Tree oil is known for its antibacterial powers and is used as an antiseptic in hand soaps and antimicrobial in dish soaps. Originating in aboriginal Australia, this oil is very powerful when applied topically as it treats cuts and prevents the risk of infection.

Witch Hazel can be substituted for rubbing alcohol because of its astringent properties causing the damaged tissues to contract and slow or stop bleeding. This will help bruise injuries to fade faster as it speeds up the recovery time of the internal damage. Witch Hazel can be applied by soaking a cotton pad or cloth and applying directly to the area.

Yarrow has been used on battlefields to treat deep puncture wounds. It has both anti-bacterial and anti-inflammatory qualities which work on the wound to both heal and prevent scarring. Yarrow is most often found in tincture or extracts form.

Swelling, Inflammation, & Arthritis

Many of the medicinal herbs available for treating inflamed joints, whether due to injury or arthritis, are taken orally. These treatments will be covered in Chapter 4. The three mentioned here are for external use only. Apply the herb extracts directly to the afflicted area for immediate results.

Aloe Vera is most commonly known for treating small scrapes and minor burns, sunburns or heat burns. The same gel you use on your sunburn can be applied to relieve the ache in your joints.

Frankincense or Boswellia is well-known to herbal medical practitioners for the plant's anti-inflammatory properties. Derived from the Boswellia tree found in India, the gum is believed to work by blocking the substances which attack a healthy joint in autoimmune diseases like Rheumatoid Arthritis. This herb is available in a topical cream form.

Eucalyptus shows up here for the tannins found in its leaves. These tannins are useful in the reduction of swelling and pain in swollen joints. You can follow up an application of Eucalyptus with a heating pad to increase the absorption into the area. This can be found in a topical oil extract. Be sure to dilute it a little with non-medicinal oil before applying directly to the skin.

Capsaicin is the active ingredient in hot peppers. For pain relief, this ingredient works to manipulate physical pain by limiting our perception of pain, triggering endorphins to release, and offering an analgesic action. The lower concentrate creams can significantly reduce arthritic pain while those with a higher capsaicin concentration works well for peripheral nerve pain. Be careful to avoid touching the eyes or other sensitive tissue when using.

Comfrey, added here for a topical treatment for broken bones, is also known as knitbone. Used as a poultice once your bone is out of a cast or if your bone area can be accessed, comfrey leaf can be used dried or fresh, steeped in a little water and oil (to prevent the leaf from sticking to the skin) and applied directly to the skin surface and covered with gauze to hold it in place. For the best results, change the poultice every couple of hours.

Skin Health, Dry & Cracked, Burns, Eczema, Psoriasis, Insect Bites and Acne

The skin is the largest organ in our body. Many of us forget to factor in the regular maintenance of this organ when we think about our overall physical well-being. Some of the following medicinal are specific to certain conditions. Be sure to test for potential allergic reactions by applying a small amount on a part of your body 12 to 24 hours prior to use on the affected area.

Aloe Vera again appears at the top of every medicinal plant practitioners list due to the gel or fluid contained within its leaves being used for centuries as a healing agent and a topical pain-reliever. Aloe can be very effective in treating psoriasis as well as all types of burns and cracked skin.

The Calendula Flower has a history of success in treating rashes and burns and certain kinds of skin ulcers. Calendula tea can be made into a compress as well as using it topically in cream form.

Comfrey roots and leaves have shown themselves useful in the treatment of rashes. Be careful though, a topical application should not last more than three days concurrently as overuse of this plant on the broken skin can lead to toxicity in the area.

The Chamomile flower, both dried and fresh, can be used in tea form as an oral rinse to treat gingivitis and mouth lesions. Externally, chamomile in cream form works to relieve itchy lesions, sunburns, and hives. Chamomile oil mixed with oatmeal in a bath is a soothing skin treatment for eczema.

Lavender, or more specifically, Lavandula angustifolia, is widely recognized for its skin healing compounds. You can find it in cream, ointment, carrier oil, and hydrosol format for almost every skin ailment there is including psoriasis, acne, and irritated skin. You can use it as a facial steam for an anti-aging treatment.

The Marshmallow root is the more common source of this plant to be found in skin and hair formulas. It is both a source of anti-inflammatory and skin-soothing agents helpful for treating eczema, burns and moisturizing dry skin.

Rose water is known for a popular scent most typically ascribed to elderly English females. They might be on to something. Roses contain antibacterial and anti-inflammatory, making them very effective in acne-prone skin. These compounds are richly effective in anti-aging care, nourishing, hydrating, and even rejuvenating skin.

Digestion

Aids for digestion are most commonly taken orally but there is one worth mentioning as an external source of comfort.

Peppermint oil contains menthol, an active ingredient in rubs and liniments. Diluting a few drops into some massage oil (sweet almond) and rubbing over the abdominal area will have a relaxing and anti-spasmodic effect on the smooth muscles of the gastrointestinal tract.

Headaches

Headaches occur for a wide variety of reasons such as tension, dehydration, fatigue, eye strain, allergies, colds, and trauma to name a few. Many of the medicinal plant sourced remedies are taken orally but there are three methods you can try externally to ease the pain. Be sure to drink water as well as trying the following.

Peppermint Oil can stimulate a marked increase of blood flowing to the forehead while soothing muscle contractions. In combination with ethanol, Peppermint Oil can reduce your headache sensitivity. You can dilute this oil with a few drops of sweet almond or coconut oil and rub directly onto your temples, forehead, and the back of your neck.

Lavender Oil is used in this context as a mood stabilizer and very mild sedative. You can place a few drops on a cotton pad or cloth and keep close by, inhaling it every fifteen minutes or so for the best effect. You can also apply the oil in the same method Peppermint oil is used.

Apple Cider Vinegar is not traditionally known as a medicinal plant. However, it is plant sourced and used for the treatment of certain ailments. Pour two cups of the vinegar into a hot bath. This will help draw the uric acid out of your body relieving tension and headaches.

Foot Care

If you are on your feet all day there is nothing like a foot bath to freshen the feet. TI prepare a foot tea, heat one gallon of water to boiling, remove from the heat and add sixteen heaping teaspoons of fresh herb. Cover, allowing to steep for twenty minutes. Strain herbs out and soak your feet. You can also stir five drops of the herb's essential oil into warm water and soak.

Catnip will relax feet that are stressed.
Chamomile, flowers, will relieve swollen feet.
Eucalyptus leaves are deodorizing and energizing.

Ginger Root will warm chronically cold feet.
Horsetail can reduce perspiration.
Juniper is an excellent anti fungal.
Loveage works as a strong deodorizer.
Peppermint can cool feet that feel overheated while energizing tired feet.

Thyme can work as both an antifungal and a foot refresher.

Eye Care

These herbs soothe tired, red eyes while softening the delicate skin around the eye itself. Take care when using herbs around the eyes. Keep the remedy as pure as possible. Below are five herbs you can create a strong decoction with, straining it twice to ensure all little bits are removed from the liquid. Use gauze of flannel to dip in the liquid and squeeze enough so that the cloth is not dripping. Lay down to apply, leaving cloth on closed eyes for fifteen minutes.

Calendula is an extremely gentle herb, very soothing to inner eye and the skin around the outer eye. Use only the flower petals for making the decoction.

Chamomile is very effective to use when your eyes are strained from overuse.

Mallow is a very useful herb. Using as a decoction around the eyes will aid with softening the delicate skin.

Mint can assist with reducing the dark circles

under the eyes. Be careful to not get any into the eye itself when using the decoction. Carefully dab on the skin itself with a cotton ball.

Rose will soothe and calm the skin around the eyes. Be careful to use only organic roses as the ones in floral markets have been sprayed with many chemicals that will harm your skin.

For Cleaning and Refreshing your Home

Lavender is a known disinfectant, mix a little oil with water and it can be applied safely to any surface. This will leave behind a scent which will calm and ease anxiety.

Eucalyptus, Tea Tree and Lavender all possess anti-bacterial properties. You can mix a few drops of all of them in some water to create a general disinfectant which also kills mold.

Lemon juice and Mint mixed together in water will provide you with sparkling windows and a fresh smell that discourages flies from hovering close by.

Chapter 4: Internal Use

Herbal medicine practices regularly use combinations of herbs designed to work together to increase effectiveness and reduce the side effects of the treatment. The synergy between the active ingredients is a common occurrence in these remedies creating the effect that the therapeutic result is greater than the sum of the ingredients involved. This can be noted in that many medicinal plants show up under multiple categories for healing.

Herbal medicines, when prescribed, are done so with the individual in mind. Dosage, combinations of remedies, and timelines are based on the individual's needs at the time. Be sure to inform yourself of the appropriate dose for your body size and lifestyle.

If you are choosing to treat your minor ailments without medical input, walking into the Natural medicine aisle of your local store can be daunting given the plethora of available options for internal treatments. Having some basic knowledge of what each herb is for can provide you with the tools for choosing the best option for your particular needs. All of the herbs mentioned here can be ingested in powder, capsule, pill, or dried or fresh form. Be careful to always read the recommended dosage on the label or follow the advice given to you by your health practitioner.

Liver and Digestion

Since the times of the Roman Empire, Artichoke has been used as a digestive herb and liver tonic. One of the stronger digestive herbs, it stimulates bile flow, improving digestion, and assisting the body in breaking down food and absorbing alcohol. Artichoke will help alleviate Irritable Bowel Syndrome (IBS), nausea, bloating, and constipation.

Dandelion is used for restoring potassium levels in the body acting as a natural diuretic and promoting a healthy digestive system. Coffee made from roasted Dandelion roots is widely recognized for detoxing the liver while also acting as a tonic. Tea made from dried Dandelion leaves can assist throughout the day in the body's excretion of excess fluids.

Ginger is an amazing warming spice that is very effective for remedying many of the body's natural functions. Introduced into Europe from China during the times of the Roman Empire, this root has a revered place in traditional Chinese medicine for over 2,000 years.

Consumption can alleviate motion sickness, nausea, expel gasses from the gastrointestinal tract, stomach cramps, and heartburn. The root can be purchased and grated into hot water to make a tea. You can incorporate it directly into your food or take it in capsule form for a more powerful effect.

Slippery Elm Bark was used by Native North Americans in poultices while European settlers used it to calm the digestive symptoms of people suffering from typhoid. The inner powdered bark of the elm tree is used today as a common remedy for acid dyspepsia, IBS, or any problem which may occur when you ingest a food that causes discomfort. The moisturizing property protects the stomach lining, easing diarrhea and intestinal cramps while flushing toxic wastes in the intestinal system. It can also be very helpful in healing the stomach lining when leaky gut syndrome occurs.

Milk Thistle, a flowering member of the daisy family, is used for digestion and to strengthen the liver. It has liver-protective powers which mean that it is effective for treating many liver disorders through maintaining the liver cells healthy and neutralizing the effect toxins have on this organ.

Peppermint, noted as an external digestive remedy in Chapter 3, returns here in oral form for relief from colic, a sluggish digestion, bloating, and gas. Peppermint oil is medically accepted as an effective treatment for IBS, as they can assist with easing the symptoms of cramps, bloating and spasms. Ingestion can take the form of infusions or teas and also in capsules for a more direct response to IBS symptoms.

Headaches, Muscle Tension

Butterbur has been effectively used for many years to treat tension headaches. The extract helps to reduce the intensity and frequency of headaches and is effective as a preventative for both adults and children. Butterbur contains both anti-inflammatory and antispasmodic qualities.

Feverfew contains a pain relieving biochemical called parthenopids which are known to limit the dilation of blood vessels on the head, a condition which can be the cause of severe headaches. Feverfew is very effective at minimizing the severity, frequency, and duration of headaches, migrants in particular.

Gingko Biloba is well known as a circulatory

stimulant specifically for the brain. It is one of the remedies for ensuring the blood stays fluid due to an anti-platelet activity property which means it is a great source for preventing headaches caused by altitude sickness.

White Willow Bark, the active ingredient in aspirin, is an excellent choice for reducing the pain that comes with tension headaches. It is highly effective and easy on the digestive system and liver making it the preferred choice for over-the-counter choices.

Devil's Claw, from South Africa, is a plant with medicine right in its roots. The plant is very good at relieving muscle tension in the neck, shoulders, and back. It can be taken in tincture or extract form.

Chamomile has 36 flavonoids, compounds which act as an anti-inflammatory. Drinking a cup of Chamomile tea will help reduce the spasms in muscles, thus alleviating pain.

Cherry Juice is very effective at minimizing muscular stress created by physical activity. Tart cherry juice will reduce pain. The antioxidants and anti-inflammatory also assist the muscles to relax to alleviate muscular tension.

Bones & Joints

All joint ailments benefit from an increased intake of essential fatty acids. This can be done by increasing your Omega 3 intake through a variety of oils available or through the supplements listed below.

Burdock Root contains sterols, tannins, and essential fatty acids. These all add up to its reputation as an anti-inflammatory. You can chop up the fresh root and use it in stir fry or make a decoction with the dried root. This herb is also available in capsule form.

Flaxseed Oil is the best option for a vegan source of Omega-3's which are essential to fight inflammation and build a healthy immune system. Note that the body absorbs the oil form much more easily than breaking down the seeds. Never cook flax or heat.

Tumeric is also an extremely effective herb for relieving joint inflammation and an effective pain remedy. It contains at least two of the same compounds found often in prescribed anti-inflammatory. Its effectiveness is the reason why it is readily used for treating cataracts, cancer, and Alzheimer's.

Stinging Nettle is another extremely effective herb used in the treatment of arthritis and gout. Anti-inflammatory properties combined with the minerals boron, calcium, silicon, and magnesium ease pain and assist in the building of a strong bone structure. Taken in leaf tea, it can help to alleviate and decrease water retention and inflammation in addition to fostering the healthy functioning of the kidneys and adrenal glands.

Licorice works very much like the body's own corticosteroids (anti-inflammatories). It can decrease the number of free radicals at the point of injury and inhibit enzyme production, a normal part of the inflammatory reaction. Licorice will also partner with the body's own release of cortisol, a naturally occurring reaction to suppress the immune system, thereby easing pain and arthritic flare-ups. It can also work to inhibit a few of the side effects of cortisol such as adrenal fatigue and resulting anxiety. Licorice can be ingested as a tea or in pill form.

Horsetail is the plant with the highest source of silica, a compound known to improve the integral tissue of the bone. It can assist with bone repair and control calcium absorption. It is best to take this in a three-week on, one-week off cycle to prevent any strain on the kidneys.

Alfalfa leaves are an excellent source of plant-based minerals essential for bone health such as calcium, magnesium, zinc, boron, and silica. The leaf is a good source of phytoestrogens, compounds used to balance out any hormonal fluctuations which can create bone ailments.

Yarrow is used in addition to the two herbs mentioned above as it increases the circulation of blood to the injured area. This is best taken in a tincture or tea form.

Comfrey, otherwise known as knit-bone, is an herb known for its rapid bone healing properties. Taken orally as soon as the injury occurs will assist in a quick recovery.

Red Clover is known to work well for people with osteoporosis due to it being a good source of phytoestrogens and minerals. Research has shown that women taking a regular supplement of red clover isoflavones developed significantly lower rates of spinal bone loss than the subjects in the placebo group.

Heart, Blood and Circulatory System

Cayenne Pepper is a favorite among herbal medical practitioners for increasing blood circulation and as a blood cleanser. As stimulate for the circulatory system, it works by dilating the blood vessels, thus increasing blood flow throughout the body. This herb can be added to your cooking or taken in pill form.

Ginger works as a nice alternative if the cayenne pepper is a bit too strong. This gentle warming herb activates blood circulation by thinning the blood. One Japanese study found it beneficial for improving the blood flow in the intestines themselves. Drinking a few cups of ginger tea each day is a nice way to stimulate your circulation system.

Prickly Ash bark is a very effective remedy for improving poor circulation of the blood resulting in cold hands and feet. The active compounds stimulate the central nervous system improving blood flow throughout the whole body.

Hawthorn has been used for years in the treatment of heart disease, mild congestive heart failure, and irregular heartbeats. The bioflavonoids occurring in Hawthorn assist in the dilation of blood vessels which protects them from free radicals, generally improving circulation throughout the whole body.

Garlic is one of the most versatile of the medicinal plants. Raw garlic contains high quantities of allicin, used to improve blood flow while also working as a diuretic to flush out excess fluids. Studies out of Britain have shown that garlic tablets increase whole body's blood circulation which results in a reduced risk of heart disease.

Cinnamon is one of the medicinal herbs that has a nice taste and is used to improve the level of blood sugar in the body and circulation. Chinese medicine doctors have accessed Cinnamon for centuries as a warming agent to assist with digestion and circulation.

Coumarin is the active ingredient which contains the compounds for thinning the blood.

Rosemary is known for improving circulation amongst those with muscle pain, sciatica, and neuralgia thereby easing muscle pain. The increased circulatory benefits include skin rejuvenation and are a good supplement for rheumatic ailments.

Yarrow, as mentioned previously, can dilate the capillaries and aids in the toning of the blood vessels themselves. It works by decongesting the capillaries, affecting the flow of blood and stimulating circulation in the body's peripheral areas. When combined with Lime Blossom and Hawthorn, Yarrow works to remedy high blood pressure and prevent blood clots from forming.

Pulmonary Circulatory System

Cinnamon shows up here again as several studies have demonstrated its positive cardiovascular effects. You can take the herb in your food, as a tea, or in pill form.

Eucalyptus's active compound is cineole. The many benefits attributed to this compound are as an expectorant, relief from coughing, soothing sinus passages and fighting congestion. Since Eucalyptus also contains antioxidants, it can also support the immune system during times of illness.

Lungwort is a plant which physically resembles its name and medicinal use. Since the 1600's, Lungwort's compounds have been effectively used to clear congestion, promote lung and respiratory tract health, and guard against organisms which adversely affect respiratory health.

Elecampane, although not well known, has been used by the Greeks, Romans, Chinese, and Ayurvedic practitioners for its soothing effects on the smooth tracheal muscles. The plant's roots contain inulin which soothes the bronchial passageways and pantolactone, an expectorant and anti-cough stimulant.

Lobelia, according to some practitioners, is the single most valuable ingredients in herbal remedies to date. Containing the alkaloid lobeline, Lobelia thins out mucus, thus breaking up congestion. Further, it stimulates the adrenal glands' response to release epinephrine, relaxing the airways, and creating easier breathing. It can also relax the smooth tracheal muscles, an active component in cold and cough remedies.

Osha Root is native to the Rocky Mountains, and North American indigenous cultures have used it for respiratory support for many years. The plant's roots contain camphor, making it one of the essential lung-support herbs. It will increase the circulation to the lungs, making deep breaths occur easily.

Peppermint (oil) can be used to promote free breathing and relax the smooth muscles along the respiratory tract. Peppermint has an antihistamine effect while menthol works very effectively as a decongestant. It is also beneficial for fighting organisms due to it being an antioxidant.

In addition to everything listed above in the Pulmonary Section, here are a few choices for dealing specifically with Hay Fever.

Tinospora Cordifolia is well known in India for relieving allergies, helping to alleviate itching, sneezing, and runny nose.

Timothy Grass (Phelum Pretense) has had many studies done regarding its effectiveness. The studies demonstrate that the pollen extract taken under the tongue can aid in the elimination of hay fever and grass pollen allergy symptoms. When injected, the herb can relieve the symptoms of seasonal allergies. Studies have also supported the belief that if given regularly to children for a few years, it can lower their chances of developing asthma.

Reishi Mushroom or the mushroom of immortality is a powerful herb used for centuries by both Japanese and Chinese medicinal practitioners. Research has shown it to be very effective as an antihistamine, controlling the release of histamines in the body.

Dental Care

For centuries, herbal products have been used in dentistry as antiseptics, antioxidants, antimicrobials, antifungals, antibacterial, antivirals, and analgesics. Medicinal herbs have been very effective in the control of microbial plaque (gingivitis and periodontitis) while aiding in the overall healing processes.

Take one teaspoon each of dried rosemary, peppermint, and lavender. Mix them together well and place in one cup of boiling water. Let steep for fifteen minutes, strain, and cool. It can also be used as a mouthwash for halitosis (bad breath).

Frankincense can be chewed in the form of a gum for promoting good oral health. The compounds contained within the oil-based resin are slowly released into the mouth and digestive tract and is beneficial for their antimicrobial, anti-inflammatory, and anti-tumor qualities. Frankincense in essential oil form is a very effective mouthwash. In powder form, the herb leads to a significant decrease in inflammatory conditions, one being plaque caused gingivitis.

Goldenseal is widely used for gum infection

treatment. Most effective as a mouthwash, when combined with Myrrh, can be a powerful antimicrobial to be used in cases of acute gingivitis.

Echinacea Root is an American Native remedy for a toothache. The root contains high levels of inflammatory.

Lamiaceae Herbs which include rosemary, mints, lavender and sage are all powerful tools for oral and dental health. They can be used in essential oil form (very aromatic) in mouthwashes and dry powder form for brushing. The leaves of the Sage plant are excellent when used fresh and applied to suppress bleeding of the gums, gingivitis, and sores in the mouth. Peppermint leaves can be chewed fresh for improvement of the breath and to alleviate inflammation of the gums.

Prickly Ash bark is a proven method to stop toothaches or any other mouth pain. It can quicken healing after a pulled or accessed tooth as it improves circulation to the mouth.

Women's health

Women have relied on medicinal herbs for thousands of years, long been known as the practitioners of herbal medicine. The accumulated knowledge from their passing on of this knowledge has brought the practice of herbal medicine to where it is today. Herbs play a significant role in providing support to a woman as she transitions through the periods of her life.

Dandelion is one herb that humans will never be without. It is a powerful tool as a diuretic for pre-menstrual bloating and combined with Stinging Nettle, works together to purify the blood. Dandelion root can be taken in the usual variety of pill forms or taken in coffee form.

Chaste Tree Berry is one of the best for providing support to a woman during her menstrual cycle. It acts as a hormone balancer through the support of the communication between the ovaries and the brain resulting in a healthy level of estrogen and progesterone in the body. This herb should be taken in tincture form.

Red Clover has the densest source of phytoestrogens which are useful when the body's natural estrogen levels are low, for example during menopause. This is useful for other menopausal symptoms such as hot flashes, night sweats, and vaginal dryness due to drops in estrogen levels. The fresh herb can be steeped in a tea and consumed as needed.

Black Cohosh flower essence is the most commonly prescribed herb for menopause. It can be combined with Red Clover to manage symptoms in addition to lifting one's mood. This root can be taken as a tincture, tea, or in capsule form.

Holy Basil (Tulsi) assists with lowering stress hormones (cortisol). It is very calming and can help with mental clarity. This is perfect for mothers who multi-task and are under a lot of stress. Holy Basil is a delicious tea and is used in tincture and capsule form as well.

There are some medicinal herbs which should never be taken with prescription medicine. The potentially fatal health effects are not something to ignore. This warning is given repeatedly and really should be actively followed. The is not to say that if you are taking prescription medication you can not ingest any medicinal herb supplements. Rather be mindful and always research the combinations before administering.

Some potentially adverse combinations include:

St. John's Wort and antidepressants – it can raise the serotonin levels in your body too much potentially leading to seizures, pregnancies in women on oral birth control and inhibited effectiveness of anti-cancer medication.

Fenugreek, can lower the blood sugar level too much and interfere with some medications for diabetes. Also it is a dangerous combination with anticoagulants (warfarin) because Fenugreek can also delay blood clotting.

Gingko Biloba, if taken with aspirin, fish oil or ibuprofen – all blood thinners, can increase the risk of bleeding. Gingko Biloba slows the clotting action of blood and can cause bleeding to occur.

Echinacea will counter act with prednisone. The steroid decreases the immune system while Echinacea stimulates it. You will receive no benefit from either if taken at the same time.

Chapter 5: Emotional Health

Medicinal herbs are often thought of as treatments for what physically ails us, boost our immune system, alleviate pain, fix our digestive problems and overall, support our physical wellbeing. It is well known that our physical body and our mental/emotional bodies are intertwined. What is happening in one will affect the other two. Both Chinese and Ayurvedic medicine practices support the theory that you cannot address an ailment without looking at all three areas of your life.

When using medicinal herbs to improve your emotional well being, look for ones that include hormone balancing properties and improve liver and gallbladder function. It is always best to work with an experienced herbal practitioner when taking herbs for mentally therapeutic purposes with deep roots. The following have been selected for their use to relieve anxiety, lift your mood, promote sleep and calmness, and to improve focus or clarify mental functions.

Sleep Aids

Lemon Balm, when consumed in tea form, has been traditionally used to treat insomnia and anxiety. It is more recently found to calm people with Alzheimer's disease who suffer from agitation.

Valerian is frequently combined with Lemon Balm, creating a mild but effective sedative for people who struggle with insomnia. It can also be taken on its own in tea form.

Catnip appears to have the opposite effect on humans that it has on cats, as humans only experience calming effects. These include relief from stress and anxiety, helps with migraines, and assists in the treatment of insomnia. You can mix the catnip with chamomile leaves to strengthen its relaxing power.

Anxiety and Stress

The herbs mentioned above are effective for responding to and improving anxiety and stress. Their only drawback is they are also effective sleep aids. The following listed here are also effective without creating drowsiness.

Lavender is a very popular herb used to calm the nerves. Essential oils can be used in a diffuser, scenting your surroundings in tranquility or placing the herb in a sachet to place under your pillow. Lavender scented creams can be applied and there are some who believe ingesting Lavender in pill form will help to reduce anxiety.

Passionflower, taken as a tea, can improve symptoms of anxiety, aviation, and irritability. It is also useful when experiencing opiate drug withdrawal symptoms.

Ashwagandha showed similar effects as those of the pharmaceutical drug lorazepam. A 2012 study showed that taking the plant extract in capsule form can significantly reduce cortisol levels without any serious side effects occurring.

Depression

St. John's Wort is the most prevalent herb used for the treatment of both anxiety and depression. It is well established as an effective anti-depressant, equivalent to those pharmaceutically created, with fewer side-effects.

Maca has been used in Peru for centuries to alleviate depression in men and women while increasing their libido. Some current research has found it very effective for treating symptoms of depression in women going through menopause. The plant is grouped according to its color, but the roots from all of the plants (black, red, cream) are helpful in treating this condition. Maca can be taken in tea or capsule form.

Ginseng has been a staple in the Chinese medicine chest for centuries. The modern-day root is derived from the American or the Asian plant. The qualities it possesses for reducing depression are that it boosts energy and improves mental clarity while reducing the symptoms of stress. These can help people suffering from reduced energy and motivation due to depression. Take note, people with bipolar disorder can trigger mania if taking ginseng.

Chamomile was studied in 2012 for its role in managing depression. The results showed that this herb does produce relief from symptoms of depression, perhaps through its action as a sleep aid. People have more energy and feel fewer symptoms.

Memory and Mental Clarity

Sage has long been known to sharpen the mind. There have been a number of recent studies to support this claim. Common as a Mediterranean culinary herb, Sage can improve mood and memory with a single dose and possibly protect memory and cognition functions in the brain.

Rosemary, another culinary herb from the Mediterranean, can improve cognitive function in low doses. Studies of the herb in aromatherapy use showed that the scent can aid memory and increase focus while reducing stress. Like Sage, Rosemary can also pick up your mood and protect your brain.

Gingko, taken in leaf extract form, is popular in Europe for treating a wide variety of conditions including memory loss and problems associated with concentration and confusion. Gingko is believed to work through the actions of increasing the blood supply, a reduction in blood viscosity and free radicals, and an increase in the presence of neurotransmitters.

Chapter 6: Growing Your Own Medicinal Herbs

Gardening and herbal medicine are both age-old practice's that have been with us for thousands of years. It is interesting to note that growing the medicinal herbs produces the same benefits as taking them. Gardening can reduce stress, bolster the immune system through exercise and fresh air, keeps your mind sharp, and helps you sleep at night. The benefits of growing your own medicinal herbs are limitless, it's no wonder so many people are turning to grow their own.

The science of gardening continues to develop and with it, the art of healing with herbs. Both have gained popularity due to concerns over our current food sources and the affordability in creating one's own food and medicine source. The availability of information on plant culture, do-it-at-home recipes for herbal remedies, and new research on the multiple uses of these remedies are creating huge potential for growth for all concerned.

In the past, it was common to devote a section of the yard for growing flowers, fruit, vegetables and herbs. These plots were an integral part of the community landscape, socializing with the neighbors over the garden fence was an integral part of a family's everyday life. Frequently, sections of these gardens were wholly devoted to the growth of plants for the purpose of home remedies.

In addition to gardens being a source of the community social fabric, they also created a link between people and nature. Habitats were created to nurture the presence of insects, butterflies, birds and snakes, all necessary for plant pollination and garden health. People kept a closer watch on the weather, relying on their joints to tell them what was going to happen. By digging up a small plot in our yard, or planting pots to set on the balcony, a medicinal herb garden is an active means of staying involved with the natural world around us.

The best advice to be given is, if you are starting an herb garden for your very first time, it is always a wise choice to keep things simple. Start small, maybe five to ten plants. Make it manageable, keep it enjoyable. That way, you will enjoy gardening, finding it pleasurable and not a chore. Plants pick up on their surroundings and beautiful, healthy gardens are built by people who love being in them.

Before you start digging and planting, there are a

few considerations to make. Obviously, if you are growing the plants in pots on a balcony, you will have fewer options in respect to sunlight and water source. One of the biggest mistakes you can make is to build your garden far away from a water source. It might seem appealing and back-to-the-earth appealing in the beginning, but hauling water, compost, and tools become very tiring over a season. Try to consider the distance from water to beds (or pots), access for a wheelbarrow to move compost in and weeds out, distance to the compost pile (if you are creating your own) and distance from your house. Of course, much of this will be pre-determined by your lot size but it is good to think of these points and create the most accessible herb plot you can.

The last considerations are sun and soil. How much sun will the plants receive in one day? Most medicinal herbs (not all, but most) would prefer to enjoy up to eight hours of sunshine a day, if not more. More sunshine will result in a higher concentration of oil inside the herb, creating a more potent plant. In respect to soil, is it acidic and filled with rocks? Clay? Sand? Some herbs prefer the Mediterranean conditions of a dry, less loamy soil with excellent drainage while other plants need a cool, shady environment. You can always amend the soil prior to planting, adding compost, peat moss, lime, and bone meal. Be sure to know once you have selected which plants you want to begin your garden with and research the soil and sun requirements prior to planting. This holds true if you are using containers.

One way to strategize the most effective garden is to draw it out. Whether it is round, oval or shaped like a kidney, pick something you will enjoy looking at. Select which medicinal herbs you would like to grow, look at their sun and soil requirements, and then research their growth patterns. Tall herbs will go in the back or the center of the bed or pot. Smaller herbs are placed at the front. If the plant likes to spread, make sure you leave enough room around for adequate growth. This map will help you remember what you have planted from year to year (some herbs are cut right back at the end of the growing season) and it is easy, as the garden grows, to forget what you have planted where.

One way to determine how healthy your soil is by looking for signs of earthworms. If it is a cool day and there are no worms just below the soil surface, you will need to add compost and a little sand to create better drainage for the plants. Organic compost will create healthy plants. Well-aged manure is very effective if it is at least a year old. Note that herbs will develop root rot easily as most of them prefer drier conditions so beware to not overwater in your zeal to get the plants growing.

Next, decide if you are going to start from seeds or buy seedlings. Seeds are less expensive to purchase. You can sprout them inside the house. Add a little organic soil to the cups inside an egg carton, a label of which seeds you have planted where, and place the carton on an old cookie sheet as the water will seep through the cardboard. Place these in a sunny and warm area of the house and in about three weeks, you will have sprouts. By planting more than you need, you will have choices of which plant looks the healthiest.

If you choose to buy seedlings to plant right away, make sure to pick the healthiest looking plants. Garden seedlings are often ready to plant the week you purchase them, so be careful to not leave them sitting in their pots for too long. Ask before you leave the store if the seedlings have been 'hardened off". This phrase refers to if the plants have been outside yet. Typically, planting occurs at a time of year where the air and ground are warmer, but it is best to acclimatize your plants to the outside by leaving them outside for a few hours a day until they are used to the temperatures. You will need to do this with the seedlings you have sprouted yourself.

Plant your seedlings at least two inches apart, more if they will grow into large sprawling plants. Mint should always be planted in a large pot as it will take over your yard in a couple of years. Oregano also has a tendency to spread out and take over. It could also be easily contained in a pot. Fill the hole with a little water, gently place the seedling in the hole, and gently press the dirt done around it. Add a little more water and take a photo – your first medicinal herb garden. It will never look this sparse again.

You can choose to plant the seeds directly into the soil. If so, make sure all risk of frost is past and the soil is reasonably warm. Keep an eye out for birds and rodents, they like to watch what you are doing then follow behind and snack on the seeds.

Medicinal plants which grow very well in pots are basil, calendula, cayenne peppers, ginger, lavender, lemon balm, mint (all varieties), rosemary, sage, St. John's wort and thyme. Note that rosemary does not enjoy being transplanted.

They can grow quite large so ensure that the space designated for them is large and they can live there forever. All of the others can be transplanted easily.

Some people plant herbs in concrete building blocks, this keeps the plant's roots warm and keeps them separate, also cuts down on the weeding. Another idea is to lay an old wooden ladder down on a bed and plant a different plant between each rung. You can plant all of the above container plants in a bed along with chamomile, garlic, feverfew, echinacea, and licorice.

Chickweed, dandelion, and plantain will show up in your yard without too much effort on your part. If you are an apartment dweller, simply visit a field far away from any roads or factories, and you will locate a large assortment of these medicinal plants growing wild.

Plants requiring a fair bit more space to grow as they get big are yarrow, valerian, mullein, burdock, and marshmallow.

Most of the medicinal plants mentioned will have the desire to spread out and take over. At the end of the growing season, ensure there is adequate space around each plant for room to grow the next season. It is very important to be a bit ruthless as healthy plants are the ones with adequate access to water and sunshine. If they are competing with others in the garden, you may lose one or two quieter herbs to more dominant varieties.

Your herbs might be in a competition for garden space but you should never feel you are competing for a gardening award. Keep in mind that if you are not enjoying gardening, you will not be reaping the peripheral benefits of having a medicinal herb garden. Harvesting your own herbs for use in your home should be a gratifying experience, allowing you to continue developing your garden and the options of remedies it can provide you with.

At varying times through the summer, you will be harvesting flowers, leaves. or roots from your plants for the creation of your home remedies. What follows is a basic guide to follow for the proper harvesting techniques to ensure you have the best quality matcrials from which to create your recipes.

You will only need to harvest the whole plant if you are requiring the roots. Otherwise, you should always only take only small amounts from each plant until your garden is well established. Then, larger harvests can be successfully undertaken as your plants will be hardy enough to sustain a larger leaf/flower loss without destroying the plant. Newer plants will only handle smaller harvesting as they are too small to sustain a whole-scale loss of leaves or flowers.

Flowerheads are prone to damage, from insects, birds, wind, or absentminded gardeners. Try to pick flowers in the morning and dry them at the first opportunity to prevent mold from growing. Any blooms that are already starting to lose their petals are past their prime and should be avoided.

Choice leaves for picking are the ones which have a healthy appearance. Biannual plant leaves should only be selected in their second year.

When you have harvested the parts of the plant you need, leaves, flowers, and seeds, store them in small cotton bags with wire frame placed inside so the leaves are not crushed or damaged.

Never mix two herbs in the same bag. They can look entirely different in your kitchen than they can in the field.

You will now need to prepare your herbs for storage as soon as possible. This is to prevent mold and mildew from growing, whereby you will have to throw out the herbs. There are many ways to preserve medicinal plants and master herbalists will each have their own method. The simplest way to store herbs is to dry them. By removing moisture from the plant, you will trap the active compounds or useful chemicals inside the plant body. This makes the plant immune to disease, mold, and other problems. Dried herbs may be stored for anywhere from three to five years without losing any of their inherent value as medicinal plants.

There are two methods for drying herbs, inside an oven or outside in the sun on a frame. The inside method is quicker, approximately one hour inside the oven as opposed to six weeks outside on the frame.

With oven drying, you will need to place your herbs on a clean, dry tray. Place a piece of aluminum foil, shiny side down, over the tray. Tuck the foil around the tray leaving only a small gap to allow moisture to escape.

Heat the oven to 150 degrees and place the tray in the oven. Take the tray out every fifteen minutes to turn the herbs over so the moisture is being evenly drawn out of the plant. When moisture is drawn out of the plant unevenly, then burning will occur. Do not let this happen. Should the plants turn brown or black, then all potency is destroyed and the plant will be useless to you.

It is very easy to over-dry or burn the plants. If you can crumble the finished, dried plant easily in your hand without it becoming powder and most, if not all, of the original color is intact, the plant is dried perfectly.

A disadvantage to this method is that herbs will lose between one-third and-one half of their potency. When the plants are dried on a frame outside, they only lose one-quarter of their original medicinal value.

For this reason, frame drying is the preferred method by experienced herbalists though it is far more time-consuming. For this option, you will require a small wood or metal box, about three-feet square, with a glass line. Line the base of the box with aluminum foil and leave a small sheltered hole for moisture to escape. Pat dry the selected herbs for drying and place on the foil, closing the lid afterward. The herbs will require turning once a day until dry, anywhere between three to six weeks.

The box should be placed in a spot with adequate sunlight and be watertight. One herb placed in the box still slightly damp will ruin the whole batch.

How you will store your herbs is determined by the method you will be using them. Ointments require powdered forms of the plant while tinctures and teas require whole roots, leave or flowers. So, a good guide to follow is that your leaves and stems are best ground, then stored while the flowers, roots, and seeds are stored whole. Be sure everything is dried thoroughly before storage.

Grinding your herbs into a powder can be done with a mortar and pestle, slower but it does allow you to decide the quality of the powder with a great deal of accuracy. An electric grinder (such as a coffee grinder) gives better uniformity to the finished product and a very fine powder.

You have now arrived at the most important step in the process. Failing to store your herbs correctly will mean you will not be able to use them. This means that all of your time and effort has been wasted.

Choose your storage room carefully. Preferably not damp, cold, or drafty nor near the kitchen as odors from cooking have been known to seep through the most airtight of containers. Never store your herbs within reach of children, they are medicine.

Choose a glass (preferably colored to keep light out), ceramic or earthenware container that is intact and airtight. Do not use anything that will allow sunlight or moisture to seep in.

Take the time to label the container carefully, as failure doing so can have fatal consequences. You should always detail the following information on the labels:

•	The date when you picked the herbs. This allows you to track its potency and renew your stocks as required.

•	The name of the herb, including the Latin and the common name.

•	The method of drying. Since potency is affected by this, it is essential that you know the method to determine the quantity for your remedies and dosage.

- The part of the herb you have stored in the container. Ground up herbs can pretty much all look the same, though the medicinal qualities of the plant vary with the part it is contained. It is very important to know which part you have stored for use.

You are now ready to begin applying your own medicinal herbs for health and symptom relief.

Conclusion

Thank you for making it through to the end of Herbal Medicine Guide for Beginners. Let's hope it was informative and able to provide you with all of the tools you need to achieve your goals whatever they may be.

The next step is to go out and identify some of the more common medicinal herbs growing wild around you. Check out the produce department and notice the variety of the herbs available, fresh and dried. Scan your supplement aisles and acquaint yourself with the varieties of remedies available, the variation in doses, and the range of ailments which can be treated.

Next, walk around your house. Do you have space for a small plot or a few containers? Start researching how much sun your plot would get in a day and what kind of soil you have. Take stock of your medicine cabinet and notice the contents. What do you seem to require the most of in your household? Maybe plan on planting a few herbs that would meet the most common of your household requirements, cuts, bruises, insomnia.

Take your paper and start building your medicinal herb bed map so that when the next growing season arrives, you are prepared to plant your very own ingredients for those herbal remedies.

Finally, if you found this book useful in any way, a review on Amazon is always appreciated!

This book belongs to a series of books about herbal medicine and how to use it to improve our life. For more information, visit www.db-publishing.com